THE COMPLETE GUIDE TO CASTOR OIL

UNLOCK HEALTH & BEAUTY REMEDIES, 20+ RECIPES & SECRETS OF NATURE'S ANCIENT HEALING ELIXIR

ESTHER CASULLI

Copyright © 2024 by Esther Casulli

All rights reserved.

No part of this book may be reproduced in any form or by any electronic or mechanical means, including information storage and retrieval systems, without written permission from the author, except for the use of brief quotations in a book review.

―――――

Book cover image officially licensed from Adobe Stock - Image #190964954

―――――

To you, the reader, who seeks not only solutions but also a deeper connection to the natural remedies that nurture your well-being—this book is for you. Your curiosity, courage, and commitment to caring for yourself inspire this work. May the pages ahead empower you with knowledge, soothe your journey, and remind you of the incredible wisdom found in nature. Thank you for trusting these words to guide your steps toward a healthier, more vibrant you.

Contents

Introduction vii

1. CASTOR OIL BASICS, MYTHS, AND FACTS 1
   Castor Oil: Myths vs. Facts 2

2. MAKING DIY HOMEMADE CASTOR OIL 6
   Method 1: Heat processing 6
   Method 2: Cold Pressing 11
   Proper Disposal of Castor Waste 11

3. USING CASTOR OIL PACKS 14
   When NOT to Use Castor Oil/Castor Oil Packs 17
   Castor Oil Packs: What You Need 18
   How to Use Castor Oil Packs 22
   How to Properly Dispose of Castor Oil Packs 25

4. FACIAL CARE 27
   Castor Oil: The Cleanser 30
   Castor Oil: Makeup Remover 36
   Castor Oil: Moisturizer 38

5. BODY CARE 43
   Castor Oil: Body Wash 43
   Castor Oil: Body Scrub 46
   Castor Oil: Body Oil 51
   Castor Oil: Body Lotion 54
   Castor Oil: Massage Oil 57

6. HAIR CARE ... 60

7. ORAL HEALTH ... 74
   So, what is oil pulling? ... 75

8. OTHER ACUTE HEALTH AND WELLNESS USES ... 79
   Castor Oil for Wound Healing ... 80
   Castor Oil Scar Tissue Massage ... 81
   Castor Oil as a Laxative ... 83
   Castor Oil Heat Packs for Abdominal Cramps ... 85
   Castor Oil for Sunburn Relief ... 87
   Castor Oil for Arthritic Pain Relief ... 88
   Castor Oil for Lash and Eyebrow Care ... 90
   Castor Oil Lip Care ... 90
   Castor Oil for Skin Treatment ... 92
   Castor Oil for Cracked Heels ... 93

9. MORE DIY RECIPES ... 96

10. GROW YOUR OWN CASTOR PLANT ... 104
    Germinating the Seed ... 104
    Indoor Care ... 105
    Outdoor Care ... 107
    Removing the Castor Plant ... 108

Conclusion ... 111
About the Author ... 113

Introduction

In the current era, there is a growing need for more natural, sustainable health, beauty, and wellness remedies. We are becoming more conscious of the products we use for our safety and environmental sustainability. Natural remedies, therefore, have gained popularity as they are safer and allow us to remain guilt-free in our quest for health, beauty, and wellness. Many natural products have become popularized over the years, but one has **stood the test of time.**

Castor oil is a versatile natural remedy from ancient Egypt to India for medicinal and beauty purposes. It is a thick, viscous, pale-yellow vegetable oil derived from pressed castor beans. The castor plant, native to the tropical climates of Africa, Asia, and Australia, is a large, fast-growing shrub that produces globe-like spiny capsules containing castor seeds/beans. Castor beans feature an elongated oval or square-ish shape with a base color of brown, red, black, brownish yellow, gray, or white.

Castor oil is a colorless to amber or pale yellow liquid with a very characteristic odor and taste, and it is obtained through mechanical pressing or solvent extraction. When taken orally, castor oil has an initially bland taste, which soon turns slightly acrid. The oil's after-taste can be nauseating, so many people tend to find ways of masking its taste. Despite its foul taste, castor oil has been used for centuries as a natural laxative, but this is not its only benefit. From health and wellness to industrial use, castor oil is extremely versatile.

As beneficial as it is, castor oil also comes with a **warning** - the castor plant and its seeds are dangerous. This is because castor beans contain ricin, a poison. This is why it is not advisable to ingest or even chew castor beans. Ricin can also be extracted from the waste material after extracting castor oil, so it is important to properly dispose of the castor plant and waste. You might remember that ricin was used as a way of murdering somebody in the Breaking Bad series. A few grains of ricin are enough to be lethal to an adult.

But, with proper handling, there is no need to fear the castor plant or its beans. Castor oil has been an absolute godsend for my family and me, especially for skin and hair care. From hair masks to moisturizers, we have incorporated castor oil into various aspects of our lifestyle. However, as we kept using it, we discovered the power of castor oil packs - a simple yet powerful remedy for pain relief, anti-inflammation, and detoxing. Castor oil is a staple in my home, and this book is my way of sharing the wonders of castor oil.

This book explores castor oil in its various forms, from growing the castor plant, making castor oil at home, and creating castor oil remedies for skin, hair, and health. I will highlight and counter the common myths about castor oil, highlight ways of making homemade castor oil, provide a buying guide for the best castor oil to use, how to make, use, and dispose of castor oil packs, and a trove of castor oil recipes for various uses. For years, castor oil's anti-inflammatory, analgesic, immunomodulatory, emollient, and detoxifying properties have been applied in ancient Egyptian, Ayurvedic, and Chinese medicine. We are finally catching on to the beauty of this oil, and this book is a beginner-friendly foray into the world of castor oil. For veteran castor oil users, this book is a reminder of the simplicity and ease of castor oil use, plus the recipes may unveil new applications.

But first things first, let's explore what castor oil is and debunk the misconceptions about this wonderful natural remedy!

Chapter 1

Castor Oil Basics, Myths, and Facts

Castor oil is a viscous, colorless pale yellow liquid that is extracted from the seed of a tropical shrub, the castor bean plant. The castor plant is native to tropical East Africa but is widely grown in the tropical climates of Africa, Asia, and Australia. The castor plant is a beautiful ornamental plant with big, bold leaves that are usually dark green, although some variants feature purple or red leaves. Red veins and petioles on castor leaves are also common. The castor plant features both male and female flowers, with the yellow male flowers appearing at the bottom of the plant and the red female flowers at the top. These vibrant colors make the castor plant great for ornamental value, but they must be monitored closely because they are highly invasive. Additionally, because of the ricin in the plant, the leaves and flowers on the castor plant can cause adverse reactions.

Fortunately, castor oil does not have the same toxicity as its plant. As evidenced by its popularity, Castor oil has been a medicinal and beauty product for centuries. Cleopatra is said to have used castor oil for ocular cleansing and to keep her eyes radiant. Presently, castor oil has become a staple in the beauty industry, with an increasing number of skin and hair care products containing castor oil. As more people become aware of its uses, castor oil has become part of the natural health and wellness space. Its analgesic properties make it a wonderful and safe pain relief remedy; its emollient properties have been capitalized for healthier hair and skin, and its anti-inflammatory properties make it a wonderful remedy for reducing inflammation and redness and general health and wellness.

However, as with all things that gain a massive following, there are claims made about castor oil, both by proponents and skeptics, that are misguided. These half-truths and misconceptions can create unrealistic expectations or misguided fear of using castor oil. So, let's explore and debunk some of the most common myths about castor oil.

Castor Oil: Myths vs. Facts

Myth 1: Castor oil is not to be taken orally

This is not true. While castor oil is not edible, consuming small amounts is beneficial for treating constipation. However, if you're buying castor oil, read the label; some castor oil is processed and should not be taken orally.

If you plan on getting castor oil for its laxative properties, choose cold-pressed organic castor oil. It's always best to be safe. Also, note that castor oil is not meant to be taken long-term.

Myth 2: Castor oil cures baldness

Castor oil's high ricinoleic acid content helps treat dandruff and scalp infections, major causes of hair loss and decreased growth. Because of its anti-inflammatory, antibacterial, and anti-fungal properties, castor oil helps relieve scalp issues and promotes blood circulation to the scalp, which improves growth.

However, castor oil cannot cure baldness, which is permanent hair loss from the scalp. It can, therefore, promote scalp health, but it cannot reverse permanent hair loss.

Myth 3: Castor oil clogs pores

With a low comedogenic score, castor oil is unlikely to clog pores. However, since most people mix castor oil with other oils, they might erroneously attribute the clogging to castor oil. It is also a low irritant and has a low allergic potential, which makes it relatively safe for topical use.

However, if you have acne-prone or congested skin, it is probably better to steer clear of castor oil. If unsure of your skin's reaction to castor oil, always do a patch test. For many people, however, castor oil is an absolute blessing in their skincare routine.

Myth 4: Black castor oil is impure

Castor oil's color depends on the method of extraction. Colorless or pale yellow castor oil is usually cold-pressed, while black Jamaican castor oil is extracted from roasted castor beans through pulverization and boiling. This is a traditional, chemical-free extraction method, and the black color is due to the ashes of the roasted seeds.

Myth 5: Castor oil packs can eliminate fibroids

Unfortunately, this is not the case. Castor oil packs are a wonderful topical application of castor oil. While they are effective in detoxing and offer relief from stomach cramps, this is not the case for uterine fibroids. The relief felt after applying castor oil packs has mostly contributed to this misconception, but don't start using castor oil packs for this reason. Many have become disappointed as these claims are too lofty.

Myth 6: Castor oil use has many side effects

This is not the case. Overusing castor oil can cause side effects or be messy. However, properly handling and using castor oil and castor oil remedies are generally safe.

Myth 7: Regular castor oil is just as good as cold-pressed castor oil

While this sentiment may seem innocent, it is a misguided belief. Cold-pressed castor oil has more nutrients and antioxidants compared to hot-pressed castor oil. Additionally, organic cold-pressed castor oil is free from chemicals. This is not always the case with hot-pressed castor oil. This is why it is always advisable to choose organic cold-pressed castor oil, especially if you take it orally.

Choosing the right castor oil is important, no matter how you plan to use it. First, always reach for the organic, cold-pressed castor oil, as you're assured it's 100% natural and safe for consumption. Second, always reach for castor oil in glass bottles. This is because, with plastic bottles, there's always the risk of plastic chemicals seeping into the oil with time. This compromises the quality of the castor oil, and it may have undesired effects. Always store the castor oil in a cool, dry place and consider the expiry date. If you prefer homemade castor oil, always ensure you don't keep it for over 12 months.

Indulging in the benefits of castor oil is a different experience for everyone. If you're looking for an indulging, adventurous journey, why not try making your own castor oil? In the next chapter, we will do just that. Turn to the next page for a step-by-step guide on making homemade castor oil.

Chapter 2

Making DIY Homemade Castor Oil

Making castor oil is, let me be honest, not for the faint of heart. While it is a simple-to-follow process, it can be messy if you're not careful. However, as you improve at making your own castor oil, it becomes a wonderful way of verifying your source of castor oil. This section includes two main ways of making castor oil - heat processing and cold-pressed.

Heat extraction is a simpler process as there is no special machinery to be bought. This makes it a common method of making homemade castor oil.

Method 1: Heat processing

This method of making homemade castor oil is popular because all that is needed is a stove, a sizable pot, a pan, a blender/grinder, spoons, and a sieve. These are usually staples in the kitchen, making this method accessible to many. However, please remember that this exercise can be time-intensive, so be prepared.

In this section, we'll explore two methods of extracting castor oil through two methods - blending and grinding.

Note:

If you're using castor beans directly picked from the tree, or you haven't yet shelled the castor beans, first start by drying the castor beans. You can lay out the beans outside in the sun to dry. However, be aware that castor beans tend to burst and throw the seeds everywhere. To prevent this from happening, first lay out the castor beans on a wide tray or place planks (if you have them) around the area where you've laid out the castor beans. Then, cover the beans with a light cloth, for example, a mesh fabric, that doesn't block the sun. This will keep the seeds from flying everywhere. Or you can shell the castor beans first and lay the seeds in the sun to dry out. Depending on how hot the sun is, this can take anywhere from 2 to 6 hours.

If you can't dry the beans in the sun, shell the beans and lay the seeds out on a baking tray, ensuring no overlap. Preheat the oven to 140°F (60°C) and pop the tray in the oven for about 7 hours. This will ensure that all the moisture content is removed.

PS: If you're drying the seeds outside, keep them away from kids or animals. As mentioned earlier, castor seeds are toxic when consumed.

Castor Oil Heat Extraction: Blending Method

- Heat a pan on medium heat.
- Once the pan is warm, add the shelled and dried castor seeds and roast on medium-high heat for about 20 minutes. Stir frequently to prevent burning. It may be hard to notice a color change, but the seeds get darker. Turn off the heat once the seeds are well roasted (not burning).
- Allow the seeds to cool for a bit, about 5 minutes.
- Transfer the seeds to a blender. If you have a lot of seeds (more than a cup), do this in batches.
- Blend the seeds to a paste, adding water intermittently to ensure you get a fine paste. Do the same for all the batches, transferring the paste into a pot.
- Once all the paste is in the pot, place it on the stove and add water while stirring until it is runny.
- Boil on medium heat for about 40 minutes, stirring intermittently to prevent the mixture from sticking to the bottom of the pot.
- Once the mixture is boiling, you have two options: First, you can choose to boil off the water from the pot. This will take a longer time, but it may work for you. When the water has boiled off, the oil will be left on the surface (If you choose this option, check the

grinding method for the next step). Second, you can choose to sieve the mixture after boiling for 40 minutes.
- Straining the mixture will help remove the chaff. Once you have sieved, preferably pour the liquid into a clear container. Place the container in the freezer for about 4 hours. The oil will rise to the top of the liquid, making it easier to scoop.
- Using a spoon, carefully scoop the oil at the top, avoiding scooping a lot of water. If possible, freeze the mixture for longer to make it even easier to scoop out the oil.
- Add the scooped oil to a pot and boil until all the water has evaporated.
- Allow the remaining oil to cool down, then strain one last time to remove all the chaff.
- Pour the oil into a glass bottle and store it in a dry, cool place away from children.
- Use within 12 months.

Castor Oil Heat Extraction: Grinding Method

- Roast the seeds on high heat for 3 to 5 minutes. Because of the high heat, you must pay attention to the seeds to prevent burning. Roasting the seeds on high heat makes them easier to grind.

- Add the seeds to a mill or grind manually using a pestle and mortar.
- Run the mill until the seeds turn into a fine paste. If you're using a pestle and mortar, this process will be much harder and time-intensive. If you have over three-quarters of a cup's worth of roasted castor seeds, instead mill or pound in batches.
- Once you have ground or pounded the seeds, add them to a pot. Add water to the pot until it covers the paste, stir slowly, and turn on the heat.
- Don't add too much water, as you will need to boil it all off. As you stir, make sure the mixture is still thick and not too runny.
- Boil the mixture on medium heat until all the water evaporates, about 4 to 5 hours, or less if you have a very small batch.
- You can stir intermittently at the beginning, but once the mixture is boiling, let it sit. Scrape the sides to prevent the sediments settling on the pot's sides from burning.
- Once the water is all boiled off, the oil will remain floating on top of the mixture.
- Turn off the heat and let the mixture cool, preferably for 24 hours. This allows the sediments to settle, making it easier to scoop the oil.

- Scoop the oil with a spoon and store it in a glass bottle or jar.

Method 2: Cold Pressing

For cold pressing, you'd need to have a cold press or an oil expeller on hand. With a price tag of over $1,000, many people don't own this machinery, making it one of the rarer ways of making homemade castor oil.

- Roast the castor seeds on high heat in a pan or a preheated oven at low heat, 140-194°F (60-90°C), for 10-20 minutes.
- After roasting, grind or crush the seeds to a paste.
- Add the paste to the oil expeller or hydraulic press. Apply pressure, maintaining a low temperature to preserve the oil's purity.
- Store the collected oil in a glass jar, preferably airtight, and use the oil within 12 months.

Proper Disposal of Castor Waste

While a 1985 paper by Okorie et al. stated that heating castor beans at 284°F (140°C) for 60 to 90 minutes neutralizes the ricin content, the waste is still toxic to young chicks. This means that disposing of castor waste needs to be undertaken with care to protect animals.

If you use the boiling method, wrap the waste tightly

in a bag and throw it in the bin as stipulated by the regulations in your area. If you have a castor plant and pick the beans from it, boil any leaves or branches that fell off the plant and the shells on medium heat for half an hour. If possible, send these to the municipal compost or put them in a bag wrapped tightly for disposal in the garbage dump.

If you use the cold-pressed method to extract the oil, you can send the waste directly to the municipal compost. Alternatively, you can boil the waste, sieve the boiled mixture, and discard it in a tightly wrapped garbage bag.

If you want to be extra careful, you can also soak the waste in bleach for 30 minutes to an hour before draining the bleach and then disposing the waste in the garbage. Always ensure that you've tightly wrapped the waste in a bag.

As you handle the waste material, make sure to wear gloves. Once the waste has been properly disposed of, clean everything you used with a lot of soap and water. Wash your hands thoroughly as well.

Castor oil assures you of its source, especially if you have your own plant. However, making your own castor oil is a time- and effort-intensive process. If you make a mistake, don't fret; it can happen to anyone. As with all new endeavors, you will definitely get better with practice. Keep at it!

On the other hand, it may be preferable for most people to simply purchase cold-pressed castor oil from Amazon or another online store.

In this chapter, we've explored various ways of making castor oil at home. In the next chapter, we'll explore one of my favorite castor oil remedies - **castor oil packs!**

Chapter 3

Using Castor Oil Packs

One of the most common uses of castor oil is in castor oil packs - simple yet effective remedies that guarantee relaxation and ease once a session is complete. From easing inflammation to improving circulation, castor oil packs provide a whole host of benefits that many natural health enjoyers swear by. Essentially, castor oil packs involve topical application of castor oil to the desired area to:

- **Alleviate pain**

Castor oil is known for its anti-inflammation properties, which greatly help reduce pain. This is especially true for joint pain, as many have touted castor oil packs as effective pain alleviation remedies. When the castor oil pack is applied to the painful joint or area, it reduces inflammation and facilitates drainage of blocked fluids, easing pain.

Many also praise castor packs for easing endometriosis pain and menstrual cramps. The ricinoleic acid in castor oil softens the muscles and drains the blockages, increasing blood flow to the area. This soothes the pain in the area as the muscles become less cramped.

- **Improve and heal the skin**

Applying castor oil packs helps to soothe issues like sunburn or bug bites. They are also wonderful for treating eczema and psoriasis, as many swear the packs have helped ease their conditions. Also, because castor oil is a moisturizer, castor oil packs can help the skin feel more supple.

- **Cleanse and detox**

Castor oil packs are also used to cleanse and detoxify the liver and intestines. This is the second-most popular use of castor oil packs. When the castor oil packs are placed over the liver and abdominal areas, the oil draws out the toxins, facilitates circulation, and alleviates muscle cramps or tightness. In addition to cleaning, the castor oil packs result in relaxation and ease, making detoxification sessions so restful that cleaning up after the session becomes a non-issue.

- **Improve gastrointestinal issues**

Castor oil's ability to help relax tight muscles makes it a wonderful remedy for reducing gastrointestinal symptoms. While castor oil is known for relieving constipation through oral delivery, this is not the only way to administer the remedy. Castor oil packs allow the gastrointestinal muscles to relax, which helps reduce constipation symptoms. While they are less effective than oral administration, they are the perfect remedy for people who can't stand the taste of castor oil or prefer not to ingest it.

When the abdominal muscles relax, this eases the pain associated with constipation and eases bowel movement. This reduces strain on the intestines, providing relief. Using castor oil packs to relieve gastrointestinal issues also relieves migraines associated with gastrointestinal discomfort.

- **Decongest the chest**

Applying castor oil packs to the chest and bronchial area can ease decongestion because of castor oil's anti-inflammatory properties.

Castor oil packs undoubtedly pack a punch, but they are not miracle cures. You will not reap the benefits of the castor oil pack with just one use. Castor oil packs work better with repeated use, so don't feel discouraged if your issue is not resolved overnight. However, you should feel better with the first session, as the castor oil packs are known for their calming and soothing effects.

When NOT to Use Castor Oil/Castor Oil Packs

While I encourage castor oil packs, they are not meant for everyone or on all issues. Do not use castor oil packs:

- During pregnancy
- When breastfeeding

(The effects of castor oil on children are unknown, so the use of castor oil or castor oil packs is discouraged. Things may change once sufficient data are obtained.)

- On recent injuries
- On irritated skin (like scratches and cuts) or on open wounds
- On open areas like the nose, mouth, eyes, or ears
- If you have a high fever
- If you have acute inflammation
- If you're on blood thinners or have a bleeding disorder
- If you have a history of cancer, chemotherapy, or radiation therapy
- If you have a history of internal obstruction or appendicitis

- If you feel gaseous

These precautions are meant to keep you safe. It is always better to protect your health than to risk it, no matter how effective the remedy may be for others. Our bodies are different, so it is better to look for safe alternatives.

Additionally, before using a castor oil pack, perform a **patch test** to ensure you do not react adversely to the oil. Simply rub a few drops of castor oil into your skin and leave it on for 24 hours. If there is no reaction, the castor oil pack should be safe to use.

Castor Oil Packs: What You Need

Castor oil packs can be easily purchased on Amazon in a variety of shapes and sizes. For example, you can purchase pre-designed and reusable packs ready for the liver, knee, and neck and for a whole host of other uses. The image below shows an example of a Sky Organics product available on Amazon. If you want to make a castor oil pack, we'll show you how to do that next.

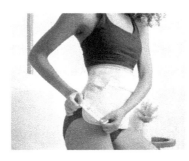

Making a castor oil pack is a simple, straightforward process. First, you need to have the following ready:

1. **A soft, clean, thick material** - Wool or cotton flannel is recommended, and it's best to choose the organic options. If you can, choose unbleached, dye-free wool or cotton flannel.
2. **Scissors (optional)** - These are used to cut the flannel into suitable sizes depending on the castor oil pack's application. Additionally, some prefer to cut the packs into individual strips instead of folding the cloth into the desired thickness. In such situations, a pair of scissors comes in handy.
3. **Glass bowl or jar (preferably with a lid)** - The size of the jar depends on the size of the castor oil pack you'll be using. However, don't think too much about this. Just choose

a bowl or jar wide enough for your hand to reach inside and deep enough to soak the flannel without making a mess. If possible, choose a glass jar solely for your castor oil packs.
4. **Tongs or gloves (optional)** - If you're uncomfortable handling castor oil with bare hands, you can use tongs or gloves when soaking the flannels and applying the castor oil packs.
5. **Hot water bottle or heating pad (optional)** - Castor oil packs can be used with or without adding heat, but for better oil absorption, adding a heating pad or hot water bottle is advised. For safety, set the heating pad on medium or low heat. If you do not own a heating pad or hot water bottle, warm the castor oil pack before applying it.

However, **don't heat the castor oil pack in a microwave.** The oil and cloth may smoke or catch fire. The best way to warm the castor oil pack is to place the glass jar in a bowl of warm water or a pot with warm water and heat it gradually, ensuring the jar doesn't touch the bottom or sides of the pot. (Make sure your jar is made of tempered glass with high heat resistance.)

You can also use a **warmed flaxseed bag**.

1. **Old clothes** - Castor oil stains fabric, so wear old clothes when using castor oil packs. Always choose clothing that you don't mind getting stained.
2. **Plastic bags** - Avoid branded plastic bags, as castor oil tends to bleed colors, contaminating the flannel. Plastic bags are used in two ways - first, to cover the surface you'll be lying on, and second, to cover the castor oil pack and prevent it from staining the heating pad or hot water bottle. Garbage bags and kitchen bags work fine, although you may need to cut them open to cover more space without wasting resources.
3. **Large towel** - Preferably, choose an old towel or one you don't mind getting stained. Place the towel over the plastic bag-lined surface you'll use for the session.
4. **Baking soda** - Baking soda is essential for cleaning up, as castor oil packs tend to be messy.

Many people consider castor oil packs "messy," but this is only when you're starting and unprepared. As you get used to the process, setting up and cleaning up afterward becomes easier. I always advise having hot water handy before and after the session, a clean rag, and a waste basket. These allow you to have a seamless clean-up in a short time.

Now that we have everything we need in place, let's explore how to set up and enjoy a relaxing castor oil pack healing session.

How to Use Castor Oil Packs

- Wear the old clothes you don't mind getting stained. Put on your gloves if you wish.
- If you're stacking your flannel strips to make the castor oil pack, place the first strip into the glass jar and pour enough castor oil over it to saturate it without dripping. Add the second strip and add more castor oil. To be safe, you can add a few spoonfuls at a time. Once all the flannel strips are soaked but not dripping, stack them on a laid-out plastic bag, making sure the pack is not dripping oil.
- If you're folding the flannel to make the castor oil pack, place it into the glass jar. Add castor oil to the flannel, ensuring it is moistened but not fully soaked. Lay out a plastic bag and place the oil-moistened flannel onto the plastic bag. Fold the flannel into the pack and add a few drops of castor oil to the side you'll place on your skin, ensuring the pack doesn't drip.

- Prepare your hot water bottle, heating pad, or warmed flaxseed bag. Remember to keep the warming pad set on low or medium.
- Cover the surface you'll be lying on with the garbage bag, then lay the towel on top. Move the wastebasket and the other items close to the bed or couch you'll use.
- If you're using the castor oil pack on your back, place the heating item on the towel where you wish to place the pack. Place a plastic bag over the heating pad, hot water bottle, or warmed flaxseed bag, then lay your castor oil pack on the bag. Lie on top of the pack, adjusting accordingly to make sure the pack aligns with the part you wish to address. Or if there's someone else with you, ask them to place the pack on your back, followed by the plastic bag and heating item (if using). However, it may be challenging to lie on your stomach for a 40+ minute session.
- For other castor oil pack sessions, simply place the castor oil pack on the desired area, cover the pack with a plastic bag, and then place the heating item on top.
- *Note:* Using a heating pad, hot water bottle, or warmed flaxseed bag is not mandatory. However, adding a heating item enhances the castor oil's absorption into the skin and amplifies its therapeutic properties.

However, you can choose not to add heat and let your body heat do the work.

- Keep the pack in the desired area for 45 minutes to an hour. You can read, meditate, or listen to music as you let the castor oil pack do its magic. You can also watch a movie, but I always suggest doing something relaxing during these sessions.
- Once your session is over, remove the heating item. Wrap the castor oil pack in a plastic bag and place it in the wastebasket next to the couch, bed, or whatever surface you're lying or sitting on.
- Mix about 3 tablespoons of baking soda in about 35 ounces (~1 liter) of warm water and clean the castor oil from your skin. If possible, place a rag in hot water mixed with baking soda when you start the session so that by the time the session ends, the rag is still warm, and you can easily wipe off the castor oil.
- Take the castor oil pack out of the wastebasket, unwrap it from the plastic bag, and place it in a glass jar or sealable plastic bag for storage. Store the pack in the fridge or a cool, dry place. You can reuse the castor oil pack about 30 times or for 2 months.

However, discard the castor oil pack if it turns rancid.
How Often Should I Use Castor Oil Packs?

When starting, feel free to use castor oil packs every other day for up to four times a week. To reuse the packs, just add a few drops of castor oil and use where desired.

If you prefer consecutive uses, you can use castor oil packs for up to three consecutive days, taking two days off before using the castor oil packs again for successive days.

For the castor oil packs to be effective, use them for multiple sessions in one area before changing to a different area. Once you feel relief, use the pack in a different area.

Note: You can have multiple castor oil packs for different areas, especially if you need different sizes for various parts. However, make sure that you pay attention to the packs and dispose of them properly when they turn rancid or after multiple uses.

How to Properly Dispose of Castor Oil Packs

Throwing away a used castor oil pack can be as easy as dumping it into a garbage bag, but I advise against this. If you're done with the pack, I suggest washing it before throwing it away. This is less messy and more environmentally conscious.

To clean the castor oil pack, soak it in a solution of baking soda and hot water for at least 20 minutes. Mix at least 4 ounces of baking soda with 2 quarts of hot water. Wring out the pack, and if you plan to reuse it, hand wash it with soap and water, then air dry. If you're planning to throw away the pack, wrap it in a plastic bag after soaking it in the hot water solution and throw it away.

Note: DO NOT wash any castor oil-stained clothing in the washing machine. Castor oil stains are impossible to remove and may transfer to other clothes. Hand wash the clothes after soaking in the hot water-baking soda solution and air dry.

If making your own castor oil pack seems too complex or messy, or **if you'd rather not make your own**, there are castor oil packs for sale online. These packs are available in various sizes depending on the application area. All you need to do is add a few drops of castor oil and apply the pack as needed. Check the packing for reuse or cleaning directions.

In this chapter, we've explored the benefits of castor oil packs and how to use them for the best results. In the next chapter, we will explore the benefits of castor oil to the skin and how to incorporate castor oil into your skincare routine.

Chapter 4

Facial Care

Skincare is an important part of our lives, as the look and feel of our skin is a huge part of who we are. The beauty industry is a multi-billion dollar industry, with people rushing to acquire products they believe will do wonders for their skin. However, many people are starting to look closely at the ingredients in the beauty products lining market shelves - from how the ingredients were sourced to the call for more transparency in "proprietary blends." As people become more intentional in their choice of skincare products, pure, ethically sourced oils have begun receiving widespread attention. Castor oil is especially gaining popularity because of its single-component composition. That is, 100% pure castor oil has no additives.

Castor oil has been used in fragrances and cosmetics since ancient Egypt, and for good reason. There is a reluctance to use pure oil on the skin because of the risk of clogged pores and breakouts. However, not all oils are the same. The comedogenic scale of oils is a 1-5 rating of how likely a specific oil is to cause acne and breakouts, with 5 being highly likely and 1 being least likely. Fortunately, castor oil has a comedogenic rating of 1, which makes it a wonderful addition to your skincare routine. Additionally, castor oil also:

- Contains ricinoleic acid, which has antimicrobial and anti-inflammatory properties. This means that it can potentially provide relief for eczema and psoriasis.
- Has linoleic and stearic acid, which, together with linoleic acid, form castor oil's amazing emollient property.
- Is stable enough that most people do not react to it adversely. However, a simple patch test is enough to determine whether castor oil is safe for you.

In addition to its host of benefits, castor oil is very adaptable. It can be used as a stand-alone product, perfect for times when you need a hassle-free, simple regimen or when you're too busy and need a quick routine. Castor oil can also be easily incorporated into other skincare routines by mixing it with existing products or creating personalized blends with other organic ingredients.

Using castor oil for your skincare routine means that

you need to choose the best product. The quality of castor oil you use will undeniably affect your skin, and you must take the utmost care for your skin's safety.

1. Always select high-quality cold-pressed castor oil. Cold-pressed castor oil retains more of its nutrients and fatty acids, providing your skin with the nourishment to foster a healthy glow.
2. Check that the castor oil is certified organic if you're not using your own homemade castor oil.
3. Castor oil should be stored in a glass jar, preferably a dark-colored glass jar. Additionally, it should be stored in a dark, dry place to minimize or prevent UV exposure. Exposure to light degrades the quality of the castor oil over time.
4. Choose packaging bottles with droppers. Droppers allow you to use just enough oil without the risk of waste. Additionally, droppers reduce the risk of contamination, which may happen if you pour excess oil back into the glass jar.

Castor oil can be incorporated into any aspect of your skincare routine, allowing you to discover what works best for you. You can incorporate castor oil in any skincare step you wish, and there are wonderful DIY recipes you can follow to create the best product to match your needs.

Castor Oil: The Cleanser

The buildup of debris, dirt, and oil on our skin as we go through our day can create unwanted issues, which is why cleansing is such an important skincare activity. Regular cleansing is important for our skin health and keeping our skin radiant. One of the more popular cleansing methods is **oil cleansing**, which is built on protecting the skin's protective oils.

Oil cleansing is a wonderful addition to any skincare routine because it protects the skin's oil barrier and maintains its pH balance. When the pH is disrupted, this exacerbates dryness, and the body compensates by producing more oil, which can cause breakouts. If you're wondering how oil cleansing can help the skin instead of causing pore blockage, it's pretty simple. By using natural plant oils, the added oil helps absorb the impurities, which are removed when you wash off the oil. Additionally, the oils tell your body that there is no need to produce more oil. This maintains and bolsters the existing oil barrier while leaving your skin clean and moisturized, depending on the oil used.

Castor Oil Cleanser Blends

Castor oil is used in oil cleansing by combining it with other carrier oils like jojoba, grapeseed, Kalahari melon, or argan. How you incorporate castor oil into your castor oil DIY cleanser largely depends on your skin type. The amount of castor oil is higher for oily skin than for dry skin. However, I advise **removing** castor oil from your cleanser blend if you have sensitive skin. Because of its astringent properties, castor oil can cause skin drying, which is detrimental to sensitive skin.

Creating a castor oil cleanser blend that matches your skin requires proper selection of the amount of castor oil in the blend and the accompanying oils.

- For oily skin, castor oil should make up 25-30% of the cleansing blend.
- For normal skin or combination skin, castor oil should make up about 20% of the cleansing blend.
- For dry to very dry skin, castor oil should make up about 10% of the cleansing blend. As castor oil can be drying, you can add a little coconut oil to counter its effects.

As you start, you can try the following recipes. However, these ratios can be altered to match your specific needs with time. This is why, as you'll notice, the measurements are just enough to make a small bath. If it works well, just maintain the ratios for larger amounts.

Blend 1 - Oily Skin
Ingredients:

- **Castor oil**

- **Core oil**: Grapeseed oil, hemp seed oil, sunflower oil, sweet almond oil, or grapeseed oil
- **Luxury oil**: Argan oil, marula oil, or sea buckthorn oil

Process:

Option 1: In a small, dark-colored glass bottle for which you have a lid or stopper, add castor oil, core oil, and luxury oil in a **ratio of 3:5:2.**

For your sample batch, this can be 3 tablespoons of castor oil, 5 tablespoons of the core oil, e.g., hemp seed oil, and 2 tablespoons of your chosen luxury oil, e.g., marula oil.

Seal the bottle with the lid or stopper and shake the mixture to combine the oils.

Option 2: If you wish to make a simpler blend, skip the luxury oil and combine castor and core oil in a **1:3 ratio.**

For a sample batch, mix 2 tablespoons of castor oil with 6 tablespoons of your chosen core oil, e.g., sweet almond oil, in a glass jar or bottle for which you have a lid or stopper.

Seal the bottle and shake to combine the oils.

Or you can choose to mix the sample batch in a small bowl and then pour the blend into a small glass bottle.

Blend 2 - Normal/Combination Skin
Ingredients:

- **Castor oil**
- **Core oil:** Sunflower oil, olive oil, apricot kernel oil, or sweet almond oil
- **Luxury oil:** Jojoba oil, argan oil, or rosehip seed oil

Option 1: In a small, dark-colored glass jar or bottle for which you have a lid or stopper (or in a small ceramic or glass bowl), mix the castor oil, core oil, and luxury oil in a **ratio of 1:3:1.**

For a sample batch, mix 1 tablespoon of castor oil, 3 tablespoons of your chosen core oil, and 1 tablespoon of your luxury oil.

Option 2: If you wish to skip the luxury oil for a simpler blend, mix the castor oil and your chosen core oil in a **ratio of 1:3.**

Blend 3 - Dry Skin
Ingredients:

- **Castor oil**
- **Core oil:** Avocado oil, sweet almond oil, olive oil, or rice bran oil
- **Luxury oil:** Rosehip seed oil, argan oil, jojoba oil, or neem oil

Option 1: In a small, dark-colored glass jar or bottle with a lid or stopper or in a small ceramic or glass bowl, mix the castor oil, core oil, and luxury oil in a **ratio of 1: 8: 1.** For a sample batch, mix 1 tablespoon of castor oil, 8 tablespoons of your chosen core oil (for dry skin, I always recommend starting with olive oil), and 1 tablespoon of your luxury oil of choice.

Option 2: For dry skin, I don't recommend skipping the luxury oil. But if you still want to, add a little coconut oil to the blend to help counter castor oil's astringent properties. Mix the castor oil, coconut oil, and core oil in a **ratio of $1/2$:1/2:5.** For a sample batch, mix $1/2$ tablespoon of castor oil, $1/2$ tablespoon of coconut oil, and 5 tablespoons of your core oil (I recommend olive oil or hazelnut oil).

If you do not wish to add coconut oil, mix the castor oil and olive/hazelnut oil in a **ratio of 1:5.**

Oil Cleansing: How To

Oil cleansing is a pretty straightforward process.

1. Start with a dry face. Do NOT wet your face before using your oil cleansing blend.
2. Start with a quarter-sized amount of the oil blend.
3. Massage it gently into your face using circular motions. Take your time to ensure the oil is absorbed into the pores, but don't rub too hard.
4. Run a washcloth under warm or relatively hot water, but not scalding. Place the warm, dampened cloth on your face and leave it on for a few seconds to a minute. The warm

cloth will help open the pores to absorb the oil and dislodge any stubborn impurities.
5. Use a warm cloth to gently wipe off the oil.
6. Wash off any remaining oil with warm water. Make sure to clean off the oil, as excess oil can clog the pores.
7. This is an optional step, but I highly recommend it. Perform a second cleanse with an active product, like an exfoliant or a gentle water-based face wash. This helps remove any lingering impurities. This is the best way to prevent clogging your pores. However, this is not always necessary if you can completely rinse off any excess oil during the oil cleanse.

As you embark on this practice, be careful not to make these **common mistakes**:

- Using cold water to rinse off the oil or dampen the washcloth.
- Applying the oil to damp skin or adding water to the oil blend. Water repels oil, which prevents the cleansing blend from effectively removing the impurities.
- Using too much oil. A quarter-sized amount should be enough, as too much oil makes it harder to rinse it off properly. Remnant oil can clog pores and cause breakouts.

Castor Oil: Makeup Remover

Castor oil can also be a simple addition to your makeup removal kit. It is an effective tool for removing oil-based and non-oil-based makeup. Its low comedogenic scale also makes it more effective for oily skin.

Castor Oil Makeup Removal Blends

Recipe 1: Castor Oil and Witch Hazel Blend
Ingredients:

- **Castor Oil**
- **Witch Hazel**
- **Vitamin E Oil**

In a small, dark glass jar or bottle or a glass bowl, mix the castor oil in a **ratio of $1^{:1:1}/_4$.** To start, mix 3 tablespoons of castor oil, 3 tablespoons of witch hazel, and $1/4$ tablespoon of vitamin E oil. Seal the jar/bottle and shake well to combine the ingredients, or use a clean glass or wood mixing stick to stir the mixture.

Store the blend in a cool, dry place away from direct light.

Recipe 2: Castor Oil and Olive Oil Blend
Ingredients:

- **Castor oil**
- **Olive oil**

In a glass jar, bottle, or bowl, mix the castor oil and

olive oil in a **ratio of 1:3.** To start, mix 2 tablespoons of castor oil with 6 tablespoons of olive oil. Seal the bottle or jar and shake well to mix the oils, or use a clean glass or wood mixing stick to mix the oils in the bowl.

Store the blend in a cool, dry place away from direct light.

Recipe 3: Castor Oil and Grapeseed Oil Blend
Ingredients:

- **Castor oil**
- **Grapeseed oil**

In a dark glass jar, bottle, or bowl, mix the castor oil and grapeseed oil in a **ratio of 1:3.** To start, mix a small batch of 1 tablespoon of castor oil and 3 tablespoons of grapeseed oil. Seal the bottle or jar and shake to mix, or stir the oils in the bowl with a glass or wooden mixing stick.

Store the blend in a cool, dry place away from direct light.

Note - If you mix the oil in a bowl, make sure to pour it into a dark glass jar with a lid for storage and to prevent contamination.

Castor Oil Makeup Removal: How To

1. Pour a quarter-sized amount of the blend in your hands and apply it to your face, or use a cotton ball, cotton swab, or cloth to apply the oil to your face. Starting with a small

amount of oil and gradually adding more will reduce waste.

The aim is to apply a generous amount of oil without dripping.

1. Leave the oil on for a few seconds, or if you can, place a warm washcloth over your face for a few seconds.
2. Gently wipe your face with a warm washcloth and dry your face.
3. To remove all the oil, you can use a gentle cleanser after.

Castor Oil: Moisturizer

Castor oil's emollient properties make it a great addition to facial moisturizing blends. When the skin is properly moisturized, it attains a wonderful, healthy glow. Moisturizers are essential to daily skincare routines as they help the skin maintain its protective barrier. Dry skin is prone to cuts, itching, and damage, which creates fine lines and ages the skin faster.

Castor oil is a natural moisturizer that traps the skin's water, preventing it from drying. With its anti-inflammatory properties, castor oil also helps soothe the skin. Adding castor oil to your moisturizing routine can take various forms, including a wonderful castor oil night serum blend, a castor oil moisturizing facial mask, and, when in a rush, a simple castor oil application before settling in for the night.

Castor Oil Moisturizing Blends

Recipe 1: Castor and Argan Oil Serum

Ingredients:

- **Castor oil**
- **Argan oil**
- **Rosehip seed oil (optional)**
- **Essential oil - lavender, tea tree, or ylang ylang**

Mix the castor oil, argan oil, rosehip seed oil, and preferred essential oil in a **ratio of 3:3:1:5 drops in a dark glass jar, bottle, or bowl.** For example, you can start with a sample of $1^1/_2$ tablespoons castor oil, $1^1/_2$ tablespoons argan oil, $1/_2$ tablespoon rosehip seed oil, and 2 drops of your chosen essential oil (I suggest ylang ylang or lavender for dry skin; tea tree for oily, acne-prone skin, and lavender for normal skin as its wonderful hydrating properties).

If you want a **simpler blend**, just mix castor oil and argan oil in a **ratio of 1:1** and add a few drops of your preferred essential oil, preferably **2 drops for every tablespoon of castor oil.**

Seal the bottle and shake to mix the oils, or use a glass or wooden mixing stick to mix the oils in the bowl. Store the blend in a cool, dry place away from direct light.

Recipe 2: Castor and Jojoba Oil Serum

Ingredients:

- **Castor oil**
- **Jojoba oil**
- **Rosehip seed oil**
- **Vitamin E oil**
- **Essential oil - lavender or frankincense**

In a dark glass bottle, jar, or bowl, mix the castor oil, jojoba oil, and rosehip seed oil in a **1:1:1 ratio**. Add **3 drops of vitamin E oil** and **2 drops of your chosen essential oil** for every tablespoon of castor oil. For example, your sample batch can include 1 tablespoon of castor oil, 1 tablespoon of jojoba oil, 1 tablespoon of rosehip seed oil, 3 drops of Vitamin E oil, and 2 drops of your chosen essential oil.

Castor Oil Moisturizing Serums: How To

1. Always perform a patch test to ensure the serum does not trigger adverse reactions or clog your pores. Apply the oil to a small part of your face and leave it on overnight. If there is no reaction, feel free to use the sample batch and make more.
2. Apply a few drops of the serum to a clean and dry face and neck and gently massage into the skin in circles. This works wonders when applied after cleansing and toning.
3. Leave overnight.

Recipe 3: Castor and Honey Moisturizing Mask
Ingredients:

- **Castor oil**
- **Honey**
- **Egg yolk**

In a glass bowl, mix 1 tablespoon of castor oil, 1 tablespoon of honey, and one egg yolk. Mix well with a glass or wooden mixing stick.

Apply the mixture generously on the face, avoiding the eyes and mouth. Let the mask sit for 15-20 minutes. Gently wash off the mask with warm water, and then apply a gentle moisturizer.

Recipe 4: Castor, Avocado, and Honey Moisturizing Mask
Ingredients:

- **Castor oil**
- **Honey**
- **Half of a ripe avocado**
- **Essential oil (optional)**

In a glass bowl, mash the avocado into a smooth paste. Add 1 tablespoon of castor oil and 1 tablespoon of honey. Add 3 drops, like lavender or tea tree, if you're using an essential oil. Mix well with a glass or wooden mixing stick.

Apply the mask generously, avoiding the eyes and

mouth. Let it sit for about 20 minutes. Wash off with warm water and apply a gentle moisturizer.

Recipe 5: Castor and Activated Charcoal Clarifying Mask

Ingredients:

- **Castor oil**
- **Activated charcoal**
- **Aloe vera gel**
- **Essential oil - tea tree, rosemary, lavender, rose, or cinnamon bark**

Mix $1^1/_2$ tablespoons of castor oil, 1 tablespoon of activated charcoal, 1 tablespoon of aloe vera gel, and 3 drops of your chosen essential oil in a glass bowl. Mix thoroughly with a glass or wooden mixing stick.

Apply the mask generously, avoiding the eyes and mouth. Let it sit for about 20 minutes, and wash it off gently with warm water. Apply a gentle moisturizer afterward.

Whether you use it as a simple cleanser, serum, or mask, there are numerous castor oil blends to try. Castor oil's adaptability has sparked its popularity in natural skin care blends, and the face is just part of it. In the next chapter, we will explore the beauty of adding castor oil to body care, where its adaptability absolutely shines through.

Chapter 5

Body Care

Castor oil's anti-inflammatory properties are amazing for reducing skin redness, and its emollience is great for maintaining a healthy glow. We sometimes focus so much on our faces that we forget that skin care is more than just the face. Castor oil can be used in body care in various ways: body wash, body oil, lotion, body scrub, and massage oil.

Understanding your skin's needs will help you determine the best way to add castor oil to your routine. Here are a few recipes to help you get started.

Castor Oil: Body Wash

Body washes are gentle cleansers that nourish and moisturize the skin, making it smooth and silky. Castor oil body washes capitalize on castor oil's wonderful emollient, antimicrobial, and anti-inflammatory properties, providing your skin with the nourishment and protection it needs. When combined with fragrant essential oils, castor oil body washes become indulgent, soaking your senses in your preferred fragrance.

Note: *Always perform a patch test to ensure the blend does not trigger any adverse reaction.*

Castor Oil Body Wash Blends

Recipe 1: Castor Oil and Raw Honey Body Wash
Ingredients:

- **Castor oil**
- **Liquid castile soap**
- **Raw honey**
- **Essential oil - lavender, tea tree, rosemary, bergamot, or chamomile.**

In a sizable glass bowl or jar, add 1 cup of liquid castile soap and $1/4$ cup castor oil. Mix thoroughly with a glass or wooden mixing stick. Add 2 tablespoons of raw honey and 10 to 15 drops of your chosen essential oil. Mix well and transfer into an empty sealable container, preferably one with a pump.

Shelf life: When stored in a cool, dry place, this body wash will last about 2 weeks.

Recipe 2: Castor Oil and Green Tea Body Wash
Ingredients:

- **Castor oil**
- **Liquid castile soap**

- **Brewed and cooled green tea**
- **Tea tree essential oil**

In a sizable glass bowl or jar, add 1 cup of liquid castile soap, $1/4$ cup of castor oil, $1/2$ cup of the brewed and cooled green tea, and 10 drops of the tea tree essential oil (feel free to use any other essential oil of your choice). Mix thoroughly with a glass or wooden mixing stick.

Pour the body wash blend into an empty sealable container, preferably one with a pump.

Shelf life: The brewed green tea shortens the lifespan of the body wash, so I advise storing it in the fridge. Use it within a week, as the potency and freshness greatly diminish after 7 days.

Recipe 3: Castor Oil and Aloe Vera Gel Body Wash
Ingredients:

- **Liquid castile soap**
- **Castor oil**
- **Aloe vera gel**
- **Essential oil - chamomile, bergamot, tea tree, lavender, or rosemary**

In a glass bowl or jar, mix 1 cup of liquid castile soap and $1/4$ cup of castor oil. Add $1/2$ cup of aloe vera gel and 10 drops of your preferred essential oil. Mix thoroughly using a glass or wooden mixing stick

Pour the body wash blend into a sealable container, preferably one with a dispensing pump.

Shelf life: The aloe vera gel in the soap is best preserved refrigerated. Store the blend in the fridge, which will last about 3 weeks.

Castor Oil: Body Scrub

Body scrubs are great skincare additions, mainly because they prevent the buildup of dead skin cells, which can clog pores and cause rough, uneven skin. Exfoliating the skin using a body scrub clears the skin of dead skin cells and other impurities. Additionally, this helps clear clogged pores, improving sebum production and the absorption of moisturizers. Frequent scrubs leave the skin feeling smoother and promote a healthier glow.

Perhaps unsurprisingly, castor oil makes a wonderful addition to body scrubs, particularly because of its moisturizing and anti-inflammatory properties. Castor oil scrubs have the added advantage of the oil's ability to absorb any excess sebum on the skin while preventing it from drying out. This allows the skin to maintain its protective layer while stimulating the sebum production.

However, you need to be cautious when it comes to the frequency of scrubbing your body. **Over-scrubbing undermines the purpose of body scrubs.** Body scrubs are meant to be a semi-frequent affair, not a daily activity. Always pay attention to the feel of your skin and how it looks. Over-scrubbing can strip your skin of its healthy glow, inflame the skin, or strip your skin of its protective layer.

- Don't scrub too hard. This might compromise the upper layer of your skin, leaving you with cuts and abrasions. Not only is this painful, but it also leaves you open to scars and impurities burrowing deeper into your skin.
- Don't scrub too often. If you have sensitive or dry skin, once a week is enough, or even once a fortnight.

Note: *As with all blends, make sure to perform a patch test. This is the best way to determine if the blend is suited to your specific needs.*

Castor Oil Body Scrub Blends
Recipe 1: Castor Oil Sugar Scrub
Ingredients:

- **Castor oil**
- **Granulated sugar**
- **Essential oil - lavender, sweet orange, vanilla, chamomile, or ylang ylang**

In a sealable glass jar or container, mix $1/4$ cup of castor and $1/2$ cup of granulated sugar. As you stir the oil into the sugar, check the consistency of the mixture. Gradually add sugar if you want a coarser scrub and more castor oil to make it less dry. Once you have your desired consistency, add 10 to 15 drops of your preferred essential oil.

Recipe 2: Castor Oil Sea Salt Scrub
Ingredients:

- **Castor oil**
- **Sea salt**
- **Essential oil - lavender, sweet orange, vanilla, chamomile, or ylang ylang**

In a sealable glass jar or bottle, mix $1/4$ cup of castor oil and $1/2$ cup of sea salt (choose the type carefully, as the size of the salt granules matters. Try to find the types with smaller coarse sea salt granules). Add the castor oil and sea salt gradually to attain your desired consistency. Add more salt for a drier mix and more castor oil for a more liquid consistency. Add 10 to 15 drops of your preferred essential oil and mix well.

Recipe 3: Castor Oil Coffee Scrub
Ingredients:

- **Castor oil**
- **Finely ground coffee**
- **Melted coconut oil**
- **Granulated sugar**
- **Essential oil - sweet almond, sweet orange, citrus, lavender, or rosemary**

In a sealable jar or bottle, mix $1/2$ cup castor oil, 1 cup coffee, $1/2$ cup coconut oil, and $1/2$ cup sugar. Make sure to mix thoroughly to achieve the desired consistency. Add a little sugar and coffee for a drier consistency and a little more castor and coconut oil for a less dry mix. Add 10 to 15 drops of your desired essential oil and mix well.

Recipe 4: Castor and Avocado Oil Scrub
Ingredients:

- **Castor oil**
- **Granulated sugar or sea salt**
- **Avocado oil**
- **Essential oil - sweet almond, ylang-ylang, citrus, bergamot, or lavender**

In a sealable glass container or jar, mix $1/4$ cup of castor oil, 1 cup of granulated sugar or sea salt, and $1/4$ cup of avocado oil. Add a little more sugar or sugar for a drier mix and a little more castor or avocado oil for a wetter consistency. Once you've achieved the desired consistency, add 10 to 15 drops of your preferred essential oil.

Recipe 5: Castor Oil Shower Gel Scrub
Ingredients:

- **Castor oil**
- **Natural shower gel**
- **Finely ground coffee**
- **Sea salt**

In a sealable glass jar or bowl, mix $1/4$ cup of natural shower gel, 1 tablespoon of castor oil, 1 tablespoon of coffee, and 1 teaspoon of salt. Thoroughly mix to your desired consistency, adding more salt or coffee for a drier consistency and a little more oil for a wetter mix.

Castor Oil Body Scrub: How To

1. Always perform a patch test to ensure the castor oil scrub blend is right for you.
2. Soak in warm water for 5 to 10 minutes; if you're in the shower, let warm water flow over your body for 5 minutes. This opens your pores, increasing the scrub's efficacy.
3. Scoop a generous amount of the scrub into your hands and gently scrub through your skin. Don't apply too much pressure or scrub too hard. If you have an exfoliating body brush or exfoliating gloves, use them. This will increase the cleansing and exfoliating impact of the scrub blend.
4. Rinse your body well and apply a gentle moisturizer (body oil or lotion) to lock in the moisture.
5. A body scrub is best done in the evenings or before bed. This allows your smooth skin and open pores to absorb the active ingredients in your moisturizer. This is also the best time for your skin's healing and repair.

Castor Oil: Body Oil

Body oils are indulgent moisturizers that do wonders for the skin and are especially effective in combating dryness or stubbornly dry spots. Hot showers, cleansing, or even a change in weather can adversely impact the skin, leaving it feeling scaly, dry, and taut. Body oils are perfect for addressing these issues, as great ones are non-comedogenic and non-greasy. Petroleum-based oils are inferior to natural body oils because of their greasy residue and clogging properties.

Castor oil's emollient and low comedogenic properties make it a wonderful addition to body oil blends. Because of its viscosity, castor oil is best added to a carrier oil, which combines the benefits of the two natural oils to create a blend that leaves the skin vibrant and supple.

Castor Body Oil Blends
Recipe 1: Castor and Almond Oil Blend
Ingredients:

- **Castor oil**
- **Sweet almond oil**
- **Vitamin E oil**
- **Essential oil of choice (optional)**

In a dark glass bottle or jar, mix castor oil and sweet almond oil in a **ratio of 1:3.** Add a few drops of vitamin E oil and 5-10 drops of your preferred essential oil. For a sample batch, mix 1 tablespoon of castor oil and 3 tablespoons of sweet almond oil. Add 5 drops of vitamin E oil and 2 to 3 drops of essential oil if using.

This should be enough to use once, and it's a great way to test various essential oils to find the one that suits you best.

Recipe 2: Castor, Evening Primrose, and Jojoba Oil Blend

Ingredients:

- **Castor oil**
- **Evening primrose oil**
- **Jojoba oil**
- **Essential oil of choice - lavender, ylang-ylang, sweet orange, citrus, bergamot, or rosemary**

In a dark glass jar or bottle, mix castor oil, evening primrose oil, and jojoba oil in a **ratio of 2:1:1.** Add in 4 - 8 drops of your preferred essential oil. For a sample batch, mix 2 tablespoons of castor oil, 1 tablespoon of evening primrose oil, and 1 tablespoon of jojoba oil. Add 4 drops of your chosen essential oil and mix well into the blend.

Enough for a single application; this sample batch will help you determine if this blend is right for you. It also allows you to change your essential oil if you wish.

Recipe 3: Castor, Coconut, and Olive Oil Blend

Ingredients:

- **Castor oil**
- **Fractionated coconut oil**
- **Olive oil**
- **Jojoba oil**
- **Essential oil of choice - lavender, sweet almond, citrus, sweet orange, chamomile, or ylang ylang.**

In a dark glass jar or bottle, mix the castor oil, coconut oil, olive oil, and jojoba oil in a **ratio of 1:3:3:1.** Add 5 to 10 drops of your preferred essential oil and mix well. For a sample batch, mix $1/2$ tablespoon of castor oil, $1 1/2$ tablespoon of fractionated coconut oil, $1 1/2$ tablespoon of olive oil, and $1/2$ tablespoon of jojoba oil. Add 3 drops of your chosen essential oil and mix well.

Creating a sample batch is important because it helps determine whether the blend is right for you. It also prevents you from wasting ingredients if you react adversely to any ingredient in the blend. Also, it can be a great way to change up the essential oils if you want.

Castor Oil Body Oil: How To

1. Body oils are best applied to a still-damp body. Apply the oil after a shower or bath so the oils can lock in moisture and keep your skin supple.
2. Applying the body oil at night allows your body to absorb the oils without the

impurities of the external world, so consider adding body oils to your nighttime routine.

Remember to perform a patch test for each blend you try. Apply the body oil to a small part and let it stay on overnight. If you don't react to it, you're good to go.

Castor Oil: Body Lotion

Many body lotions are on shelves, making it difficult to find good ones that match your needs. There is also a rise in natural-based lotions, but sometimes, these fail to be 100% natural, or there is uncertainty about how the ingredients are sourced or processed.

Fortunately, you can make your own body lotion, which gives you greater control over the ingredients you choose and allows you to eliminate chemicals used to preserve the ingredients in mass-produced products.

Body lotion is essential to body care because of its moisturizing properties. It prevents us from walking around with dry, ashy skin and smells wonderful. DIY castor oil body lotion blends keep your skin moisturized while allowing your skin to benefit from the active natural ingredients mixed with castor oil. Additionally, your chosen essential oil allows you to indulge in the scent of your choice.

Castor Oil Body Lotion Blends

Recipe 1: Castor Oil and Lavender Moisturizing Lotion

Ingredients:

- **Castor oil**
- **Olive oil**
- **Shea butter**
- **Beeswax**
- **Lavender essential oil**

In a double boiler, mix $1/4$ cup of castor oil, $3/4$ cup of olive oil, and $1/2$ cup of shea butter. Heat the mixture over medium heat, stirring occasionally. Once the mixture melts into a liquid consistency, add 2 tablespoons of grated beeswax and 10 - 15 drops of lavender essential oil. Mix thoroughly.

Allow the mixture to cool slightly, but don't let it solidify. Pour the mix into a blender and blend at high speed until light and creamy, about 2 minutes.

Transfer the lotion blend into a sealable container.

Note: If you don't have a double boiler, melt the mixture in a heat-safe bowl and place it over simmering water.

Recipe 2: Castor Oil and Coconut Oil Lotion
Ingredients:

- **Castor oil**
- **Coconut oil**
- **Cocoa butter**
- **Almond oil**
- **Beeswax**

In a double boiler, mix $1/4$ cup of castor oil, $3/4$ cup of coconut oil, and $1/2$ cup of cocoa butter. Warm the mixture on medium heat until it melts, stirring occasionally. Add 2 tablespoons of almond oil and 2 tablespoons of grated beeswax to the mixture and mix thoroughly.

Let the mix cool down slightly, but don't let it solidify. Pour the melted blend into a blender and blend on high speed for about 2 minutes until light and creamy. Pour the blend into a sealable container and use as desired.

Note: If you don't have a double boiler, melt the oil mix in a heat-safe bowl over simmering water.

Recipe 3: Castor, Shea, and Oat Milk Lotion
Ingredients:

- **Castor oil**
- **Shea butter**
- **Oat milk**
- **Essential oil of choice - vanilla, lavender, rosemary, or sweet almond**

In a double boiler, mix 1 cup of castor oil and $1/2$ cup of shea butter. Warm on medium heat until the oil blend melted, stirring occasionally. Pour $1/2$ cup of oat milk stir, then add 10-15 drops of your preferred essential Mix the blend thoroughly.

llow the mix to cool slightly, but don't let it solidify. he mixture into a blender and blend quickly for minutes until light and creamy.

Pour the blend into a sealable container.

Note: If you don't have a double boiler, warm the oil mix in a heat-safe bowl over simmering water.

Castor Oil Body Lotion: How To

1. Apply the body lotion on clean skin, preferably after a shower or bath. Make sure to generously apply the lotion on drier areas to keep them moisturized.
2. You can transfer a little lotion into a travel-size bottle and carry it throughout the day as hand lotion.

Always perform a patch test to ensure the lotion does not trigger any adverse reaction.

Castor Oil: Massage Oil

A simple massage is enough to help us destress, unwind tight muscles, and sink into relaxation despite our busy days. Massage oils make the experience much more invigorating as we indulge more senses in the massage session. Adding oil massages to your routine helps to declutter your mind while allowing your skin to enjoy the oil's innate goodness.

Castor oil massage oils are moisturizing, adding a wonderfully silky feeling to your skin. The oil's scents help indulge more senses depending on the essential oils used. Massage oils can be used for full-body sessions or when you need to relax a certain body part. Adding massage oil to warm bathwater is also a wonderful way to destress and decompress.

Because of its anti-inflammatory and emollient properties, castor oil makes a great addition to DIY massage oil blends.

Castor Oil Massage Oil Blends

Recipe 1: Simple Castor and Essential Oil Massage Oil

Ingredients:

- **Castor oil**
- **Essential oil of choice - you have the freedom to use two or three**

In a glass bowl, mix 2 tablespoons of castor oil and 3-5 drops of your preferred essential oil. This batch is enough to apply to a problem area or a sore spot on your skin. If you wish to make more, just add castor and essential oils in the same ratios.

Recipe 2: Castor and Almond Oil Massage Oil

Ingredients:

- **Castor oil**
- **Almond oil**
- **Essential oil of choice - you can choose to mix two or three if you wish**

In a glass bowl, mix 1 tablespoon of castor oil, 3

tablespoons of almond oil, and 3-6 drops of your preferred essential oil. Mix thoroughly with a glass or wooden mixing stick. This batch is enough to apply to a problem area, and you can make more if you wish, maintaining the same ingredient ratios.

Feel free to substitute almond oil with coconut or olive oil.

Castor Oil Massage Oil: How To

1. If you're planning to treat a problematic or sore area, apply a generous amount of the massage oil blend to the desired area and gently massage, adding pressure if necessary.
2. If you plan a full-body massage, make more oil using the ratios provided.

You can always warm the oil before use by placing a heat-safe bowl with the oil in a pot with hot water. This allows the oil to heat gradually.

Always perform a patch test before committing to the massage oil blend.

Castor oil's adaptability is not confined to facial and body care. Many have attested to its wonders in hair care, from scalp care and nourishment to hair growth. In the next chapter, we will explore the wonderful impact of adding castor oil to hair care, including a few DIY recipes.

Chapter 6

Hair Care

Hair care is important and not just for aesthetic purposes. The state of our hair impacts our mood, well-being, and self-confidence, even if we don't realize it. This is why we panic when we lose hair strands in the shower, have an inflamed scalp, or experience stubborn dandruff. With the abundance of hair care products on the market, finding one that meets our needs can become frustrating.

The hair care space, just like the skincare space, has witnessed a significant shift toward more natural remedies. People are becoming more selective in their chosen products, from shampoos to hair dyes. This is because the chemicals present in synthetic products are being exposed for their adverse effects on the scalp, skin, and even body. This means that people are becoming more willing to spend a few extra minutes whipping up their own DIY hair products instead of spending countless hours and hundreds of dollars trying new products to find which ones work for them.

And fortunately, this has highlighted how we can capitalize on castor oil's versatility for our needs. Castor oil is a wonderful addition to hair care because of its moisturizing and nourishing effect. In addition to improving hair shine, castor oil is wonderful for scalp health. Its antifungal and antibacterial properties help reduce dandruff; its emollient properties keep the scalp moisturized without clogging the pores; its anti-inflammatory properties help improve blood circulation in the scalp, nourishing the scalp and hair follicles.

As with its skincare diversity, castor oil can be added to various aspects of hair care, from a cleansing shampoo to a nourishing hair mask. In this chapter, we'll explore some castor oil DIY recipes to help you keep your scalp and hair healthy.

Note: *Always perform a patch test before committing to any recipe. This will help you determine if the ingredients are safe.*

Castor Oil Shampoo Blends

Note: Making your own castor oil shampoo blend is simple and straightforward. However, because of the natural ingredients, I always advise making small amounts for one-time or two-time use. We tend to store shampoo in the bathroom, which is humid. This decreases the shelf life of your DIY shampoo, and depending on the ingredients, mold can begin developing in the shampoo.

The degrading quality can cause unwanted side effects or adverse reactions, so making small one-time-use batches just before use is better.

Recipe 1: Castor Oil and Manuka Honey Nourishing Shampoo

Ingredients:

- **Castor oil**
- **Manuka honey**
- **Liquid castile soap**
- **Olive oil**
- **Coconut milk (organic; homemade if possible)**

In a glass bowl or jar, mix 3 tablespoons of castor oil, $1/2$ teaspoon of Manuka honey, 2 teaspoons of liquid castile soap, $1/2$ teaspoon of olive oil, and 2 teaspoons of coconut milk. Using a glass or wooden mixing stick, thoroughly mix to get a smooth consistency.

Recipe 2: Castor and Tea Tree Clarifying Shampoo

Ingredients:

- **Castor oil**
- **Tea tree essential oil**
- **Liquid castile soap**
- **Vegetable glycerin**
- **Distilled water**

In a glass bowl, mix 4 tablespoons of castor oil, 4

tablespoons of liquid castile soap, 1 tablespoon of vegetable glycerin, and 2 tablespoons of distilled water. Whisk the mix thoroughly for a smooth consistency. Add 8-12 drops of tea tree essential oil and mix well.

Recipe 3: Castor and Carrot Seed Oil Nourishing Shampoo

Ingredients:

- **Castor oil**
- **Liquid castile soap**
- **Carrot seed oil**
- **Maple syrup**

In a glass bowl or jar, mix 1 teaspoon castor oil, $1/2$ cup liquid castile soap, 1 teaspoon carrot seed oil, and 2 tablespoons maple syrup. Gently mix to a smooth consistency.

Recipe 4: Castor Oil and Apple Cider Vinegar Soothing Shampoo

Ingredients:

- **Castor oil**
- **Apple cider vinegar**
- **Liquid castile soap**
- **Tea tree essential oil**

In a glass bowl or jar, mix 4 tablespoons of castor oil and 4 tablespoons of apple cider vinegar. Mix well and add $1/2$ cup liquid castile soap and 10-15 drops of tea tree essential oil. Gently mix until you achieve a smooth consistency.

Castor Oil Shampoo: How To

1. Apply the shampoo to wet hair, generously applying to the scalp and hair roots.
2. Gently massage the shampoo into the scalp to encourage circulation.
3. Lather the shampoo through the hair and rinse thoroughly with warm water.

Note: *If the amount suggested in the recipe is insufficient, just double the ingredients. However, always ensure that you make enough for two uses. Natural ingredients like honey, coconut milk, and maple syrup can easily accelerate mold growth in the product if the shampoo is not stored properly.*

Castor Oil Hair Mask Blends

Looking for a way to incorporate castor oil's tremendous benefits into your hair care routine but feeling skeptical of adding oil to your shampoo? Worry not. You can still have castor oil as part of your routine and keep your beloved shampoo.

A hair mask is an infrequent deep treatment that helps your hair and scalp absorb active ingredients. It is wonderful for hydrating, nourishing, and strengthening dry, damaged hair. Hair masks are simple to apply, and their consistent use results in stronger, healthier, and less frizz. Castor oil mask blends allow you to enjoy the benefits of castor oil's moisturizing, anti-inflammatory, and antimicrobial properties.

Note: *The recipes in this section feature natural organic ingredients that cannot be left out for too long. Make these hair masks fresh before use, and dispose of any leftovers after you're done.*

Recipe 1: Castor Oil and Avocado Hair Mask
Ingredients:

- **Castor oil**
- **Ripe avocado**
- **Coconut oil**
- **Essential oil of choice (optional)**

In a glass bowl or jar, mash 1 ripe avocado (small- or medium-sized; if you have a large avocado, use half) to a smooth consistency free of lumps. Add 2 tablespoons of castor oil, 1 tablespoon of coconut oil, and 5 drops of your chosen essential oil if using. Mix well to a smooth consistency.

Recipe 2: Castor Oil and Yogurt Hair Mask
Ingredients:

- **Castor oil**
- **Plain Greek yogurt**
- **Raw honey**

In a glass bowl or jar, mix 2 tablespoons of castor oil, 3 tablespoons of Greek yogurt, and 1 tablespoon of raw honey. Mix thoroughly to form a smooth consistency.

Recipe 3: Castor Oil and Shea Butter Hair Mask
Ingredients:

- **Castor oil**
- **Shea butter**
- **Jojoba oil**
- **Coconut oil**
- **Essential oil of choice (optional)**

In a double boiler, mix 4 tablespoons of castor oil and 4 tablespoons of castor oil. Warm the mixture on medium heat until the shea butter is melted through. Stir occasionally to ensure the oil is mixed well. Remove from heat and allow to cool slightly before adding 1 tablespoon of jojoba oil and 2 tablespoons of coconut oil. Mix thoroughly and add 5-10 drops of your preferred essential oil if using. Mix well until you have a smooth consistency.

Recipe 4: Castor, Coconut, and Egg Hair Mask
Ingredients:

- **Castor oil**
- **Coconut oil**
- **Egg yolk**
- **Raw honey**

In a glass bowl or jar, mix 3 $^1/_2$ tablespoons of castor

oil, 1 egg yolk, and $1/2$ tablespoons of raw honey. Whisk the mixture to a smooth consistency.

Recipe 5: Castor Oil and Aloe Vera Hair Mask
Ingredients:

- **Castor oil**
- **Aloe vera gel**
- **Tea tree essential oil**

In a glass bowl or jar, mix 2 tablespoons of castor oil and $1/2$ cup aloe vera gel to a smooth consistency. Add 3 drops of tea tree essential oil and mix thoroughly.

Castor Oil Hair Mask: How To

1. Apply the hair mask blend to dry or damp hair. I recommend damp hair as it is easier to spread the blend. Make sure to apply generously from the root to the ends.
2. Gently massage the blend into your scalp using your fingers or a wide-toothed comb to promote circulation and coat all hair strands.
3. Leave the mask on for about half an hour (some like to keep the mask on overnight, but this is not a must). Tie your hair into a bun if possible.
4. For deeper penetration, cover your hair with a shower cap or plastic wrap.
5. Rinse your hair thoroughly with lukewarm water, not hot water. The cooler temperature

will seal your pores, which helps seal in the moisture.
6. Shampoo and condition your hair as usual, preferably with natural products, to avoid buildup.

Note: *If you have dry or damaged hair, applying a mask once a week will help hydrate and moisturize your hair. If you have oily hair, a mask a few times a month will be sufficient. (Make sure to do a patch test before committing to a blend to ensure you don't have any adverse reaction to any ingredient.)*

More Castor Oil Hair Blends

Recipe 1: Castor and Jojoba Oil Pre-Swim Conditioner

Ingredients:

- **Castor Oil**
- **Jojoba Oil**

In a dark glass dropper bottle, add 3 tablespoons of castor oil and 1 tablespoon of jojoba oil. Seal the bottle and shake vigorously to mix.

How to use: Using the dropper, add a few drops of the blend to your scalp and massage gently and comprehensively to ensure your entire scalp is well-oiled. Add a few drops to your palm and run your fingers through your hair strands, from root to end.

After swimming, rinse your hair with warm water,

shampoo it, and condition it with gentle products to remove any residual oil.

Recipe 2: Castor, Coconut, and Rosemary Scalp Massage

Ingredients:

- **Castor oil**
- **Coconut oil**
- **Rosemary essential oil**

In a heat-safe bowl, add 3 tablespoons of castor oil and 1 tablespoon of coconut oil. Add the bowl to a pot or bigger bowl with hot water to gradually warm up. Once the oil is warmed, remove the bowl and add 3 drops of rosemary essential oil to the blend. Stir the blend thoroughly.

How to use: Apply the blend to your scalp using a dropper or your fingertips. Massage the oil blend into your scalp, adding more as needed. Gently massage your scalp for 5-10 minutes. Rinse off the oil with warm water and gentle shampoo.

You can also leave the oil on overnight, wrapping your hair to avoid staining your clothes or bedding. In the morning, rinse off the oil and follow your usual shampoo and conditioner ritual.

Recipe 3: Castor Oil and Rosemary Hair Elixir
Ingredients:

- **Castor oil**

- **Rosemary essential oil**

In a dark-colored glass dropper bottle, mix 4 tablespoons of castor oil and 2 tablespoons of rosemary essential oil. Seal the bottle and shake vigorously to mix the blend.

How to use: Apply the oil blend to your scalp using the dropper. Gently massage the oil into your scalp for a few minutes to promote circulation. Leave the oil on overnight, making sure to wrap your hair to avoid staining your clothes or bedding. Rinse off in the morning with warm water and use a gentle shampoo to clean off any oil residue. Condition your hair as usual.

Recipe 4: Castor, Argan, Coconut, and Jojoba Hot Oil Treatment

Ingredients:

- **Castor oil**
- **Argan oil**
- **Coconut oil**
- **Jojoba oil**
- **Vitamin E oil**
- **Tea tree essential oil**

In a double boiler, add 1 teaspoon of castor oil, 1 tablespoon of argan oil, 1 tablespoon of coconut oil, and 1 teaspoon of jojoba oil. Warm the mixture on low heat until it is warm to the touch but not scalding (If you don't have a double boiler, add the oils to a head-safe bowl and place it over boiling water.). Remove from heat and allow the oils to cool slightly. Add 4 drops of Vitamin E oil and 5 drops of tea tree oil. Stir the blend until the oils are well mixed.

How to use: Make sure the oil is warm but not hot. Apply a few drops of the oil blend to your scalp using a dropper or fingertips. Gently massage the oil into the scalp, ensuring your entire scalp is well nourished. Leave the oil on for at least half an hour, or you can leave it on overnight. A heat cap can open your pores and improve oil absorption. If leaving the oil on overnight, wrap your hair to avoid staining your clothes or bedding.

Rinse off the oil with warm water, using a gentle shampoo to remove any residue. Condition your hair as usual.

Recipe 5: Castor and Argan Oil Pre-Shampoo Treatment

Ingredients:

- **Castor oil**
- **Argan oil**

In a heat-safe glass bowl or a double boiler, mix 3 tablespoons of castor oil and 1 tablespoon of argan oil. If using a glass bowl, warm the oil by placing it over hot water. If using a double boiler, warm the oil on low to medium heat.

How to use: Using a dropper or fingertips, apply the oil generously to your scalp. Gently massage the oil into your skin for a few minutes. Leave the oil on for at least half an hour. Use a heat cap to help open the pores for better oil absorption. If you plan to wash your hair immediately, apply more oil to your hair strands. If leaving the oil on overnight, wrap your hair to avoid staining your clothes or bedding.

Before rinsing your hair in the morning, coat your hair strands with the oil blend and leave on for 5-10 minutes. Rinse your hair with warm water and use a gentle shampoo to remove any residue. Condition your hair as usual.

Castor oil is a hair care ally as its diversity makes it great for protective and restorative measures. Castor oil pre-shampoo blends protect the hair and scalp from being stripped of natural oils while cleaning with shampoo; as a hair mask, it helps moisturize the scalp and nourish damaged, dry hair; scalp massage blends help increase circulation in the scalp while infusing the hair with active ingredients; as a pre-swim conditioner, castor oil helps protect the hair from the harsh chemicals in the swimming pool or salt in the sea or ocean; and as hot oil treatment, castor oil blends moisturize and nourish the hair.

We've explored the wonders of castor oil's diversity but have yet to exhaust its uses. Amazing, right?

In the next chapter, we'll explore castor oil's application in oral health. Because the next chapter features internal use, make sure to only use cold-pressed, 100%

natural and organic castor oil that's safe for internal use. Preferably, choose castor oil that's safe for ingestion in small amounts as it will come in handy a lot more times than you think. Now, let's explore the link between castor oil and oral health.

Chapter 7

Oral Health

Using oil for oral health has become popular recently, but this does not mean that the movement is a fad or a trend that will be forgotten. On the contrary, including oil in oral health is based on an ancient Ayurvedic practice dating back as far back as 5000 years. While the ancient practice was more spiritual than hygienic, this does not make it any less effective.

Oil pulling started as a way of using oil to draw out spiritual energy through the gums. However, practitioners derive various other physical benefits depending on the oil used. For example, using castor oil for oil pulling may require putting up with its acrid taste, but it's wonderful for reducing oral inflammation because of its anti-inflammatory properties. This partly explains the rising popularity of castor oil for oil pulling.

Oil pulling is essentially based on the premise that

the oil will help remove stubborn oil-soluble impurities and particles, improving oral health. While many skeptics disregard this claim, it is not entirely unfounded. Oil pulling, in conjunction with standard oral hygiene practices, helps reduce plaque and total bacterial count. Oil pulling is even more beneficial for people with oral devices and appliances, e.g., dentures and retainers.

So, what is oil pulling?

Oil pulling involves swishing oil in your mouth for a few minutes, similar to how we use mouthwash. This practice removes oil-soluble particles and impurities and addresses gum inflammation or other oral issues for some. Oil pulling is also a great way to clean oral devices and appliances, as the oil helps absorb impurities that latch onto the crevices and are resistant to brushing or standard oral cleaning.

Using castor oil for oil pulling is beneficial in three main ways:

- Because of its anti-inflammatory properties, oil pulling with castor oil helps reduce oral inflammation, especially gum inflammation. This helps to reduce the risk of infection and inflammation-related pain.
- Castor oil's antifungal properties are particularly helpful to people who have dentures. The Candida albicans fungus

resides in our mouths in small quantities. However, the fungus can become problematic for denture wearers as they adhere to the surface and oral tissues. The fungus thrives and overgrows if the dentures are improperly cleaned or stored. This poses a great risk to the denture wearer, as their risk of developing denture stomatitis increases.

Castor oil's antifungal properties hinder the growth of fungi, decreasing the chance of developing denture stomatitis. For non-denture wearers, castor oil hinders the development of fungi in the oral tissues, improving general oral health.

- Castor oil's antimicrobial and antibacterial properties may not heal existing mouth problems, like cavities, but they help slow down further damage. Oil pulling with castor oil results in lower gingival and plaque scores and reduced oral bacterial count.

These castor oil benefits make it an excellent choice for oil pulling. Oil pulling is a simple exercise requiring no fancy additional devices. So, whether you have any oral devices or are just looking to improve your oral hygiene, you should give oil pulling a chance.

Oil Pulling: How To

Make sure to purchase high-quality castor oil, preferably cold-pressed. Check that it is safe for oral use.

1. Measure 1 tablespoon of castor oil (about 15 ml) and put it in your mouth.
2. Swish the oil around in your mouth for a few minutes. Many recommend 15-20 minutes, but even 5 minutes is enough. You are always allowed to start with a few minutes and build up the time as you get used to the taste and practice of swishing oil.
3. Spit the oil into a napkin and throw it into a garbage can or waste bin. DO NOT spit the oil down the sink. The oil will clog the pipes over time.
4. NEVER swallow the castor oil. Because it is a stimulant laxative, swallowing the oil will result in some pretty inconvenient side effects.
5. Brush your teeth and floss as usual.

Note: Oil pulling is **not a substitute** for normal oral hygiene practices. It should accompany regular brushing and flossing. Oil pulling is a complementary oral hygiene practice.

Tip: If you don't have time to dedicate to oil pulling, add it to your other routine, like swishing as you make coffee or prep your shower or bath.

And that's basically it for oil pulling. It is best practiced regularly, especially if you have any oral devices. With brushing and flossing, you will have less plaque, no bad breath, and fewer chances of contracting oral infections. In the next chapter, we'll explore how castor oil can be added to general health practices. It can be an instrumental addition to our general health and wellness routines. Let's see how!

Chapter 8

Other Acute Health and Wellness Uses

Castor oil's uses are not only confined to beauty purposes. In addition to hair care and skin care, castor oil has been used to help address various health and wellness-related issues. The most well-known castor oil used is to address constipation because of its property as a stimulant laxative. Castor oil is also used to treat small wounds, burns, and cramping pain because of its emollient and anti-inflammatory properties. However, there needs to be care and intentionality when dealing with castor oil. Many assume there may be no side effects because castor oil is a natural product; although the side effects are rare, other considerations must be made.

In this chapter, we will explore the various castor oil applications that help improve our well-being while addressing some of our life's pain points.

Castor Oil for Wound Healing

Open cuts are common enough that we all have home remedies for faster healing and to prevent scars. Adding castor oil to the wound healing kit is worth considering. However, medical practitioners caution against using castor oil on fresh cuts or burns at home. This is a valid concern; castor oil must be mixed with other ingredients before being used for new wounds. Additionally, improper application of castor oil to a new wound can be detrimental to the healing process. And it's always better to be safe than sorry.

However, adding castor oil to wound care is perfectly alright as the wound starts to scab over. When castor oil is applied to a healing wound, its emollient property helps to trap moisture in the skin. This prevents the skin from drying out and promotes tissue growth. When the skin is well moisturized, this also prevents sores from developing. Castor oil also seals off the wound, which prevents infection.

How To Use:

1. Always ensure that the castor oil you are using is clean. This is why I recommend using castor oil in a bottle with a dropper and a Q-tip or wearing a clean latex glove for application.
2. Using the dropper, place a little oil on the Q-tip or glove and carefully apply it over the

wound. Make sure to apply a small amount to avoid dripping.
3. If the wound is covered by clothing, make sure you dab off any excess oil to minimize staining your clothing.
4. Always clean the wound before applying castor oil to avoid trapping dirt and debris.
5. Dispose of the Q-tip or gloves. Always use a new one for every application. Seal the castor oil and store it in a cool, dry place away from direct sunlight. You can also store the castor oil in the fridge.

Castor Oil Scar Tissue Massage

Scars are a natural part of healing; scars come in all shapes and sizes. However, scars can be a source of physical and emotional discomfort. Scar tissue can be hard and unyielding, which tends to pull the skin, limiting mobility depending on the scar's location. Scar tissue massage is a remedy to ease the discomfort by softening the scar tissue to allow more mobility and relieve discomfort. Castor oil is a popular part of scar tissue massage because, for some people, the regular use of castor oil in this way has significantly reduced scar tissue. This has led to the widespread belief that castor oil can help eliminate scars. While this may have been true for some, it is not always the case. Everyone's scars are different, and the changes experienced can be similar or very diverse.

I always recommend accepting the changes as you experience them. Lofty ambitions may lead to disappointment and a mistaken conclusion that it is a fad. That being said, let's explore how to use castor oil effectively for scar tissue remedy.

How To Use Castor Oil As A Scar Tissue Massager

1. Thoroughly clean the scar to remove debris, dirt, and natural oils from the area. It is enough to wash the area with a soapy, warm washcloth and rinse it off with a wet washcloth.
2. As before, I recommend using castor oil stored in a bottle with a dropper. It is always advisable to use clean castor oil, and a dropper greatly minimizes any chance of contamination.
3. Since you'll use your fingertips for this practice, you can wear gloves or ensure your hands are clean.
4. Place a pea-sized amount of castor oil on your fingertips. Apply the oil gently on the scar, making sure the entire scar is coated in oil.
5. Gently massage the scar tissue with your fingertips, exerting enough pressure to rub in the oil effectively. However, you should not cause yourself any pain.

6. Massage the scar tissue consistently for 3-5 minutes or up to 10 minutes if you wish.
7. Once you've completed the massage, place a warm towel over the area and let it sit for 10-15 minutes. This helps open the pores to absorb the oil deeper into the scar tissue.
8. If you wish, you can wipe off the oil or let it sit as you go about your day.
9. If you have more time, apply a castor oil pack to the scar after the massage session. Let the pack sit for 30 minutes to an hour, placing a heat source over it.

Perform the castor oil scar massage regularly for the best results. It is not an overnight miracle, but it does make a difference with time, so don't give up.

Castor Oil as a Laxative

Castor oil's use as a laxative is perhaps its most known purpose, with many advising caution against administering this seemingly harmless oil carelessly. There are many types of laxatives, and their categorization is based on how they function. Castor oil is a stimulant laxative. Stimulant laxatives trigger movement in the intestines, prompting the intestinal muscles to push out the stool.

The intestinal movement can sometimes cause abdominal cramps, so I always recommend using castor oil as a laxative when you can rest and relax at home. Because it is a stimulant laxative, castor oil works fast, so you need to take it when or after you're settled in the comfort of your home.

Apart from the abdominal cramps, other side effects include burping, nausea, and diarrhea (which is to be expected).

How To Take Castor Oil As A Laxative

1. Ensure that the castor oil is safe to consume - preferably cold-pressed high-quality castor oil.
2. Measure out 1 tablespoon (about 15 ml).
3. If you can withstand the acrid taste of castor oil, you can just swallow the oil. However, since the taste and aftertaste can be overwhelming, I recommend adding the castor oil to a glass of fruit juice after refrigerating it for about an hour or so.
4. Do not take it before bed since it works fast (within 6 to 12 hours).

Caution: Taking castor oil as a laxative should not be done too regularly. If your issue has not been resolved within a week, seek medical help. Additionally, there are other cautions to take:

- Do not administer castor oil to a child 12 years or under without medical consultation.

- Do not administer if over 60 years old to prevent exacerbating bowel issues.
- Do not take castor oil regularly for a long time, as it may decrease intestinal muscle tone, resulting in severe constipation.
- Do not administer if pregnant.
- Consult a healthcare professional before taking castor oil if you have high blood pressure, diabetes, and heart disease.
- Do not administer if you have symptoms of appendicitis, irritable bowel syndrome, undiagnosed rectal bleeding, or intestinal blockage.
- Do not administer if you're allergic to stimulant laxatives.

The cautions highlighted above are to keep you safe. Always honor your limits. There's no heroism in recklessness.

Castor Oil Heat Packs for Abdominal Cramps

This is a simple remedy that you can choose if you can't create a castor oil pack and still need relaxing relief from the pesky cramps. It's a simple castor and essential oil blend that promotes relaxation as your pain fades into the background.

Heat Pack Blend

Ingredients:

- **Castor oil**
- **Essential oils - peppermint, eucalyptus, and lavender**

In a small glass bowl, mix 2 tablespoons of castor oil and 1 tablespoon of each lavender oil (feel free to substitute any essential oil for your preferred one). Mix thoroughly with a glass or wooden mixing stick. Place the bowl over a pot or bigger bowl of hot water to warm the oil if you want to.

How To Use Castor Heat Pack Blend

1. Dip a wool or cotton flannel into the bowl to soak it in oil (make sure you use a small piece, just enough to cover your lower abdominal area). Alternatively, slowly drizzle the oil over the flannel to soak it.
2. Cover the flannel with a plastic wrap or a soft cloth you don't mind staining.
3. Place a heating pad or hot water bottle over the plastic cover or cloth and let it sit for 20-30 minutes.
4. Clean the area with a warm washcloth. You can dispose of the oil-soaked flannel in the bin (make sure to wrap it securely) or store it in an airtight container in the fridge for the

next session. Just add a few drops of castor oil and your preferred essential oil.

Castor Oil for Sunburn Relief

Castor oil's anti-inflammatory and emollient properties have made it a natural sunburn remedy. Sunburnt skin can feel painful and uncomfortable and can be unpleasant to look at. Fortunately, castor oil is a simple remedy that can help ease the skin's healing process.

Castor oil can be used alone or with raw honey or aloe vera for sunburn relief.

Process 1 - Castor Oil

1. Making sure your hands are clean, measure out a pea-sized amount of castor oil and apply it gently to the sunburnt area.
2. Add more oil if needed. The aim is to cover the area with castor oil without the oil dripping.
3. Keep applying to clean skin until it has healed.

Process 2 - Castor Oil and Raw Honey

1. In a small glass bowl, mix 1 tablespoon of castor oil and 2 teaspoons of raw honey (or Egyptian honey). Make sure to mix well.

2. Using a dropper or the end of your mixing stick, add a pea-sized amount of the blend to your fingertips (make sure your hands are clean).
3. Apply the blend to the desired area, adding the blend as desired.
4. Store any remaining blend in the fridge and use within 24 hours. After that, ensure to make a new blend.

Process 3: Castor Oil and Aloe Vera

1. In a small glass bowl, mix 1 tablespoon of aloe vera gel and 10 drops of castor oil.
2. Using the end of your mixing stick or a clean wooden spoon, add a dime-sized amount of the blend to your palm (ensure your hands are clean).
3. Dip your fingertips into the blend and apply it to the desired area, coating it gently but thoroughly.
4. Store any remaining blend in the refrigerator and use within 24 hours. After that, always make a new blend until the skin is healed.

Castor Oil for Arthritic Pain Relief

Castor oil's anti-inflammatory property comes in pretty handy when dealing with joint pain, particularly arthritic joint pain. When applied, castor oil does not dry out, keeping the skin around the joint well-nourished and supple. Castor oil helps promote blood flow to the joint, reducing joint stiffness

and inflammation.

Castor oil can be used to relieve arthritic pain in two ways.

How To Use Castor Oil For Pain Relief

Process 1: Castor Oil Packs

1. Castor oil packs are great for joint pain relief as they give the castor oil time to do its magic.
2. Apply the pack to the joint and relax for 30-40 minutes.

Process 2: Castor Oil Wraps

1. If you're short on time, a castor oil wrap is the way to go.
2. Using a dropper, generously apply castor oil to the desired joint. Ensure the area is well coated by the oil, but don't let it drip.
3. Wrap the joint in a gauze bandage and leave it on for a few hours.
4. Alternately, cover the joint with a warm towel until it cools. Remove the towel, but don't wash off the oil just yet.

Castor Oil for Lash and Eyebrow Care

Castor oil nourishes the scalp and promotes circulation, making it a popular hair care product. It results in healthier, stronger hair. Because of this, castor oil has also been promoted as a wonderful product for eyelash and eyebrow care. Testimonies have ranged from longer, fuller lashes to healthier, fuller eyebrows, fueling the use of castor oil as an essential hair growth elixir.

How To Use Castor Oil For Lash and Eyebrow Care

1. Using a dropper, add a little castor oil to a Q-tip. Gently run the castor oil Q-tip over one eyebrow. Add castor oil to the other side of the Q-tip and run it over the other eyebrow.
2. Do the same for the lashes, being careful not to poke yourself in the eye. Apply the castor oil to both the upper and lower lashes.
3. Always use a clean part of a Q-tip to apply each side. This prevents the transference of debris and dirt.
4. Apply the castor oil regularly. The results will be evident in due time.

Castor Oil Lip Care

Dry lips can be a pain. Lip care should be undertaken regularly for smooth, soft lips. Castor oil is a wonderful addition to lip care because of its emollient properties. Additionally, it promotes circulation and further nourishes the lips for that healthy, beautiful glow.

For lip care, here is a simple DIY recipe for a lip balm.

Castor Oil Lip Balm Recipe

If you use lip balm tubes or pots, have 10 tubes or 5 pots on hand.

Ingredients:

- **Castor oil**
- **Organic virgin coconut oil**
- **Organic beeswax (grated or pellets)**
- **Vitamin E oil**
- **Essential oil of choice (optional) - lavender, peppermint, sweet orange, or rose.**

In a double boiler, add 2 tablespoons of beeswax and melt on low heat. Once melted, add 2 tablespoons of castor oil and 4 tablespoons of coconut oil. Mix the blend with a wooden stick, maintaining the double boiler's low heat. After 4-6 minutes, remove the blend and let it cool.

When the blend has cooled slightly, add 20 drops of Vitamin E oil and 15 drops of your preferred essential oil (you can mix two essential oils if you wish; just keep the cumulative amount to 15 drops). Mix the blend, and while still warm and melted, pour into the tubes or pots

(If the blend hardens before pouring, warm slightly). Once hardened, seal the tubes and pots.

Note: If you do not have a double boiler, place a heat-safe glass bowl in a pot of hot water.

Castor Oil for Skin Treatment

Castor oil can be an effective remedy for a variety of skin issues, including ringworms, dry skin, itching, athlete's foot, warts, and pigmentation. Its antifungal, emollient, and antimicrobial properties help relieve dryness while also fighting off fungal infections, making castor oil a wonderful natural remedy.

However, it's best to note that using castor oil to resolve pigmentation issues will take time to see results. So, don't expect an overnight miracle. Keep using the oil regularly, and the results will become evident in time.

How To Use Castor Oil For Skin Treatment
Process 1: General Use

1. Using a dropper, add a drop or two of castor oil to a cotton ball. Apply the castor oil to the desired area, making sure to use a new cotton ball if you're applying it to multiple areas (e.g., if you have an athlete's foot and need to apply it between your toes).
2. Leave the oil on for a few hours before washing off with warm water.
3. For the best results, apply at least twice daily.

4. If the area is covered or cannot be left open, cover the spot with a clean cotton cloth after applying the castor oil.

Process 2: Ringworm Treatment

1. In a small glass bowl, mix $1/2$ tablespoon of castor oil and 1 tablespoon of organic coconut oil.
2. Using a dropper, add a few drops of the blend to a cotton ball and apply it to the affected area (you can also dip the cotton ball in the oil). If you have multiple ringworms, use a clean cotton ball.
3. Cover the area with a cloth, place a cotton pad over it, and secure it with a band-aid.
4. Leave on for 6-8 hours. Alternatively, apply the blend at night and leave it on overnight.
5. Apply daily for the best results.

CASTOR OIL FOR CRACKED HEELS

Cracked heels are uncomfortable, and you cannot afford to ignore them as the fissures tend to grow deeper, which may turn into painful wounds. Having dry heels is not a novel thing, as this can happen because of wearing sandals, weather changes, or even just having cold, dry skin.

Castor oil is a great remedy for cracked heels because

of its thickness, which means it takes time to be absorbed, and its emollient properties. Its antimicrobial and antifungal properties help keep infections at bay, especially if the cracks are somewhat deep.

How To Use Castor Oil For Cracked Heels

1. Soak your feet in warm - plain or soapy - water for 10-15 minutes. Gently scrub with a loofah or exfoliating gloves.
2. Pat your feet dry.
3. Apply castor oil to the feet and coat the heels generously.
4. Put on a pair of socks. Choose socks that you don't mind getting stained. The socks will help keep the feet warm and contain castor oil stains.
5. Do this daily, gently scrub your feet to avoid breaking the already fragile skin.
6. Once healed, moisturize the heels regularly, especially if you have dry skin.

Castor oil's versatility is a godsend, as your bottle of castor oil will always have a function. This is why I always recommend storing your castor oil in a bottle with a dropper. This minimizes contamination, allowing you to use your castor oil whenever needed without buying a new bottle.

We have finally explored how to use castor oil, but this is not the end. The next chapter features 10 more DIY recipes that I think you'll find interesting. So, turn the page and see what's in store!

Chapter 9

More DIY Recipes

As promised, here are some DIY recipes to put your castor oil to good use!

Recipe 1: Castor Oil Mocha Lip Scrub

Ingredients:

- **Castor oil**
- **Granulated white sugar**
- **Cocoa powder**
- **Coffee grounds**
- **Peppermint oil extract**

In a small glass bowl, mix 1 tablespoon of castor oil and 2 tablespoons of sugar. Add 3 drops of peppermint oil extract and mix well. In a different container, mix $1/2$ teaspoon of coffee and $1/2$ teaspoon of cocoa powder. Add the mix to the castor and sugar blend. Mix well.

If the mixture is a bit runny, add more sugar. Pour the mixture into a lip balm pot or glass jar.

It is safe to use for about 2-3 months if you keep it dry. If water gets into the scrub, make a new blend.

Recipe 2: Castor Oil Body Butter
Ingredients:

- **Castor oil**
- **Raw mango butter (or shea butter, illipe butter, or cocoa butter)**
- **Jojoba oil (or organic coconut oil)**
- **Essential oil of choice - lavender, sweet orange, chamomile, or vanilla**

In a double boiler, mix $1/4$ cup castor oil, $1/2$ cup raw mango butter (or raw butter of choice), and $1/4$ cup of jojoba oil (or carrier oil of choice). Melt the blend on medium heat. If you don't have a double boiler, melt the mix in a heat-safe bowl and place it over simmering water. Once the oils are melted and well mixed, remove them from heat and allow them to cool slightly.

Add 10-15 drops of your desired essential oil. Mix the mixture until smooth and creamy using a hand mixer or whisk. Store in a sealable container.

Recipe 3: Castor Oil Lash and Eyebrow Serum
Ingredients:

- **Castor oil**
- **Sweet almond oil**

- **Vitamin E oil**

In a small glass bowl, mix 1 tablespoon of castor oil, $1/2$ tablespoon of sweet almond oil, and 5 drops of Vitamin E oil. Pour the oil into a sealable glass bottle with a dropper or a mascara tube (ensure the tube is cleaned and sanitized beforehand).

Use a mascara wand to apply the serum to your lashes and a clean cotton ball or Q-tip for your eyebrows. Apply daily before sleep for the best results.

Recipe 4: Castor Oil Peppermint Soothing Heel Balm
Ingredients:

- **Castor oil**
- **Shea butter (or cocoa butter)**
- **Olive oil (or organic coconut oil)**
- **Beeswax (optional)**
- **Peppermint essential oil**

In a double boiler (or heat-safe bowl placed over simmering water), melt 2 tablespoons of castor oil, 2 tablespoons of beeswax (if using), 1 tablespoon of shea butter, and 2 teaspoons of olive oil. Warm the blend over medium heat and mix well. Remove from heat and allow to cool slightly. Add 15-20 drops of peppermint essential oil.

Pour the blend into a sealable container and let it solidify before sealing it. Apply the balm and wear socks to make the blend work its magic. Apply daily before bed for the best result.

Recipe 5: Castor Oil Turmeric Pain Relief Blend
Ingredients:

- **Castor oil**
- **Turmeric powder**

In a small bowl, mix 2 tablespoons of castor oil and 1 teaspoon of turmeric powder to form a paste.

Using your fingers (ensure your hands are clean), apply the paste to the aching joint. Leave the paste for 20-30 minutes, then rinse with warm water. If you must move around, wrap the area with a bandage gauze after application.

Recipe 6: Castor Oil Green Tea Hand Cream
Ingredients:

- **Castor oil**
- **Green tea (brewed and cooled)**
- **Beeswax (pellets or grated)**
- **Shea butter**
- **Vitamin E oil**
- **Essential oil of choice (I recommend chamomile)**

In a double boiler (or heat-safe bowl placed over simmering water) on low heat, melt 4 tablespoons of castor oil, 4 tablespoons of grated beeswax (or pellets), and 4 tablespoons of shea butter. Once fully melted and mixed, remove from heat and allow to cool slightly. Gradually add the cooled green tea (do not surpass 4 tablespoons) as you stir until the mixture is at your desired consistency. Add 10 drops of vitamin E oil and 5 drops of your preferred essential oil. Mix well and pour the blend into a sealable container.

Allow to cool completely and solidify before sealing the container. Use as desired.

Recipe 7: Ginger Infused Pain Relief Castor Oil Pack
Ingredients:

- **Castor oil**
- **Grated ginger root**

In a double boiler (or heat-safe bowl placed over simmering water) on low heat, warm 1 cup of castor oil, but don't let it boil. Remove from heat and add $1^1 1/2$ tablespoons of grated ginger to the warm oil, letting it infuse for 5-10 minutes or until the oil is warm enough to be safe on the skin.

Dip your cotton or wool flannel into the blend to soak, then place it in the desired area. Cover the flannel with plastic wrap, then place your hot water bottle or heating pad over the plastic wrap. Let the pack sit for 30-40 minutes.

I recommend disposing of this infused pack after every use because of the ginger root.

Recipe 8: Peppermint and Arnica Pain Relief Blend

Ingredients:

- **Castor oil**
- **Beeswax pellets**
- **Olive oil (or organic coconut oil)**
- **Peppermint essential oil**
- **Arnica oil**

In a double boiler on low heat (or heat-safe bowl placed over hot water), melt 4 tablespoons of castor oil, 2 teaspoons of beeswax pellets, and 1 tablespoon of olive oil. Once the blend is completely melted, remove it from heat and let it cool slightly. Add 20 drops of peppermint essential oil and 15 drops of arnica oil. Pour the mixture into a sealable container and seal it once it is completely cooled.

Apply a small amount of the blend to the desired area and gently massage until absorbed. Because castor oil's absorption is slow, always start with a small amount and add more if needed.

Recipe 9: Castor Sweet Almond Beard Oil
Ingredients:

- **Castor oil**
- **Sweet almond oil**
- **Jojoba oil**
- **Tea tree essential oil (or other essential oil of choice)**
- **Vitamin E oil**

In a small glass bowl, mix $1/2$ tablespoon of sweet almond oil, $1/2$ tablespoon of jojoba oil, 5 drops of castor oil, 3 drops of tea tree essential oil, and 3 drops of Vitamin E oil. Store the blend in a small glass bottle with a dropper.

Apply a drop or two after showering while your beard is still damp. Massage the oil into the skin gently.

Recipe 10: Massage Oil Candle
Ingredients:

- **Castor oil**
- **Soy wax**
- **Shea butter**
- **Cocoa butter**
- **Fragrance oil of choice - make sure it is candle- and skin-safe**

In a double boiler on low heat, melt $1^{1}/_{2}$ tablespoons of soy wax and $1^{1}/_{2}$ tablespoons of cocoa butter. Once melted, remove from heat and add the shea butter. Stir the mixture constantly until all the shea butter has melted. Add $3/4$ teaspoon of castor oil and 1 teaspoon of fragrance oil (e.g., love spell, lavender, bergamot, etc.).

Pour the mixture into a shallow glass container (since you'll be pouring out the wax, using a tall container will worsen the tunneling), ensuring that the wick you choose is primed with soy wax and not paraffin wax. If the blend doesn't harden after a few hours, add a little more soy wax to the blend (make sure to melt the blend on low heat).

This has been a fun, practical chapter. And just like this chapter, the next one is for those with a little adventure in them. In the next chapter, we will explore the basics of growing your own castor plant.

Chapter 10

Grow Your Own Castor Plant

Growing your own castor plant is a journey on its own. In this chapter, we will explore what you need to witness the beauty of the castor plant while giving yourself a chance to live through the castor oil lifecycle - from seedling to oil.

Caution: Always wear gloves when handling the castor bean plant.

Germinating the Seed

Castor oil thrives in warm climates, so it's best to time the germination period with the average last frost date. Because of the castor plant's toxicity, it will be easier to germinate your own seed than to find a seedling. If you live in a warm climate, you can plant the seeds directly in the garden or outside. However, for those in colder climates, you must grow the castor plant indoors for about 6-8 weeks. So, start the germination and indoor period about a month or two before the warm season.

- First, soak the castor seeds in warm water (or compost tea) for 24 hours before sowing.
- To facilitate sprouting, ensure the seeds are in a warm environment. You can plant them in a plastic container with a cover, keeping the seeds in the container long enough to sprout before replanting them in a pot. You can also plant them in the pot, but ensure you cover it with plastic wrap. Alternatively, you can place the pots in a large plastic bin and keep it covered.
- Ensure that you sow the seeds 1" to $1^1/_2$" deep.
- Keep the soil moist, and ensure that the pots or bins are placed in the warmest place in the room (you can use a heat mat).
- Once the seeds sprout, they will grow pretty fast. So, ensure that you transplant them to a bigger pot (2"-4") once they sprout.

Indoor Care

The castor plant tends to grow fast, and you need to be responsive to its needs if you want the plant to grow out instead of just high.

- Castor plants require plenty of light to grow, and light passing through the window is not enough. Get a grow light to ensure the plant grows strong instead of tall and weak. Keep the light on for 14-16 hours a day, adjusting the light as the plant grows.
- Keep the plant in the warmest part of the house and ensure that there is enough air flow in that area.
- Always keep the soil moist, not wet or soggy. And never let the soil dry out. Once you water the plant, ensure that you dump any excess water in the trays.
- When the first set of true leaves appears, you can add fertilizer. Choose an organic fertilizer or compost tea, making sure to start with a weak dose.
- As the castor plant grows, watch out for weak sprouts. You can choose to thin out the plant, especially if you planted multiple seeds in a single hole. However, don't pull out the sprouts. Rather, cut the weak sprout off at the base.
- Once the plant grows to 3"-4" tall, it is time to move it outside or replant it.

Outdoor Care

Castor plants are vibrant and bold, but their toxicity means that you must be extra careful with where you grow them. First, ensure that your chosen location is inaccessible to children and animals. Second, the castor plant is invasive. So, you must keep trimming the flowering spike regularly to control its growth and sometimes pull out larger plants for disposal.

- Before permanently transplanting your castor plant, you must slowly adjust it to the outdoors. Place the plant outside for a few hours daily, preferably in a shady area.
- Slowly reposition the plant to get more direct sunlight, gradually increasing the time you keep it outdoors.
- After a few weeks, the plant should be "hardened" enough for the outdoors.
- If you're replanting them, space them out properly (about 36" apart) to give them room to grow. Overcrowding stunts the castor plant's growth. With enough space, the castor plant leaves get to grow to their signature massive sizes.
- Ensure that you choose a warm location with lots of sunlight and mild winds.
- To ensure that the plant grows out and not just tall, pinch the growing tip (for a bushy

castor plant, pinch the main growing tip when the plant is about 2" tall).
- Ensure that the soil drains well and the plant has enough sunlight, water, and fertilizer.
- Harvest the spiky seed pods when they appear. This keeps the plant under control while also encouraging flowering and production. Alternatively, you can prevent the formation of seeds by cutting off the flowers before they mature. This way, you maintain even better control of the plant's growth.

And that's it! Once the castor plant has taken root outside and is thriving, just keep on top of the seed pod harvesting and keep children and pets away from it.

Removing the Castor Plant

- If you wish to get rid of the castor plant for whatever reason, pull them out by the roots if possible. If the plants are too big, cut them down (as close to the ground as possible) and dig out the roots. Make sure to wear protective clothing when removing the castor plant.
- Place the plant and roots in heavy-duty garbage bags. I recommend double bagging.

- Call your local waste management office (or any relevant office) and inquire about the proper disposal procedure for toxic plants. Make sure to follow the instructions provided.
- Keep monitoring the area where the castor plant was to ensure there are no more regrows. If the castor plant sprouts, pull it out by the roots and properly dispose of it. Repeat until there are no more regrows.
- **DO NOT** burn or bury the castor plant as a way to dispose of the plant.
- After handling the castor plant, thoroughly wash your tools and protective clothing. Then, shower or wash your hands and any exposed skin with soap and lots of water.
- If your castor plant grows out of control, call a professional landscaper or a pest control service. Seeking professional help maybe your best course of action.

The castor plant may come in handy if you plan on making your own castor oil, but I recommend considering the implications of planting the castor bean plant in your garden. Unlike many ornamental plants, the castor plant can have serious ramifications if mishandled. So, if your plant growing record has been less than stellar or you have kids and pets, I advise against growing your own plant.

Safety is always the priority!
And... that's it for this castor journey!

Conclusion

Throughout this book, we have explored the wonders of castor oil. Despite its inherent toxicity, castor oil has grown into a popular natural beauty and wellness tool. While it comes with various cautions, castor oil is pretty much harmless when handled with care.

First, never consume castor beans. Second, always ensure that you handle the castor plant with gloved hands and, when necessary, protective clothing. Third, always adhere to the proper dosages. Finally, always choose organic, cold-pressed castor oil for your recipes.

Adding castor oil to your routine can take various forms, including skincare, hair care, beard care, lash care, oral care, and even pain relief. The recipes highlighted in this book are fun, simple ways of infusing castor oil with the benefits of other oils to make application easier or add a pleasant scent that matches your preferences.

So, don't just write off castor oil if one recipe doesn't

work out. The book's measurements are low, allowing you to switch out the complementary ingredients and experiment with your blends. This book is a starting point, a launch pad from which you can gain a little experience and confidence to create your signature blends.

So, dip into your castor oil and create the blends, packs, and wraps you need or want. All you need is a little time and motivation. Feel free to reach out if you have any questions, corrections, or recipe recommendations. I'm always looking for new castor oil recipes to try.

And... **thank you so much for making it to the end!** I appreciate it. I am glad you enjoyed this book or found any value within its pages. I hope you'll take a moment to review the book. This will help the book reach more people new to the castor oil journey or aficionados looking for new recipes to try out.

Again, thank you for reading this book. I hope your castor oil journey is as fruitful as mine :)

Yours,
    Esther Casulli

About the Author

Esther Casulli is of Italian-American descent, and is an emerging author of wellness & beauty self-help guides. This is Esther's first book.

www.ingramcontent.com/pod-product-compliance
Lightning Source LLC
Chambersburg PA
CBHW020005130125
20280CB00013B/1173